D1738368

BRAVE HEARTS

3 RULES FOR MEN
WITH THE COURAGE TO LOVE

Cameron Draeco

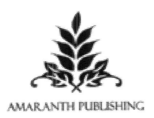

AMARANTH PUBLISHING

CONTENTS

To my mother, Florencia
Thank you for putting me on the path towards my mission.

To my children, Alexi and Franco
Thank you for giving me the support and strength to stay true to my
mission.

INTRODUCTION

HI! I'M BEWILDERED.

MY MARRIAGE OF THIRTY years ended a couple of years ago, and it left me bewildered. Because within those three decades, we never fought. And when I say never, I mean never. Not a raised voice. Not a door slammed. Not a single F-word in either one of our faces.

We raised two loving, responsible children who grew up believing we were one happy family. But beneath the masks we wore as a couple, there lurked a quiet pain and emptiness. It was a slow unraveling of the ties that bound us together. A barely perceptible erosion of the ground on which we walked. After years of holding up the weight of our hidden sadness, the foundation that held up our marriage collapsed.

I had given it my all—or so I believed—and yet it still came to an end. And that is what left me bewildered. How could things have gone wrong between us—two decent, peace-loving people who at one time had believed we had enough love to keep us together till death do us part? I needed answers so I could heal from my past and brace myself for the future. I talked with my friends and extended family, and I was stunned to discover that many of them felt trapped in their own version of a miserable marriage—that's if they hadn't separated already. All of them wanted to hear my story; even those who were happily married. Besides wanting to give me emotional support, I could tell they wanted to learn from what I shared. Either to bolster what they had or get some catharsis from it.

I stayed for decades in a kind of relationship that many were still enduring. Some of them were even worse off because each day was a constant exchange of criticism, contempt, defensiveness, or thick walls of stone-cold silence.

I may have left a marriage and ended up bewildered, but they were already bewildered while still living in theirs.

So I read and researched and took courses in psychology, cognitive behavioral therapy, and emotion-focused relationship counseling. I learned of data released in 2019 from a survey conducted by the Pew Research Center on marriage and cohabitation in the U.S. It showed that love, indeed, is the reason most couples chose to marry. 90% of respondents cited love as their reason for tying the knot. 73% of those living with a partner also gave love as their reason for moving in together.

Yet despite that, the statistics as of 2022 show that somewhere between 40% and 50% of first marriages in the U.S. end in divorce. As for second marriages, the divorce rate is even higher at somewhere around 65%. And based on what I've learned from secret heartaches shared by friends and family as well as my own, it definitely doesn't mean that those who stay married are happy where they are.

Now that I'm a certified relationship counselor—and having been exposed to both population-wide numbers as well as private and personal stories—the resounding conclusion I couldn't escape is: Love is not enough.

So what else do we need then? As vital as that information is, it's not something we're formally taught. School dealt with reading, 'riting, and 'rithmetic. There's not much in there about romance and relationships.

Age-wise, in physical terms, I'm on the brink of retirement. Mentally, I'm a new student in the school of life and the psychology of relationships. Emotionally, I'm discovering parts of myself that are only now maturing.

I learned my lessons the hard way. And through this book, hopefully you won't have to.

Preface

Who This Book is For

THIS BOOK IS DEDICATED to men in love. Those brave enough to admit it to themselves. Profess it to the woman they love. And most of all, demonstrate their love for that woman without apology or shame to other men.

Admittedly, it contains a lot of generalizations about men and women in romantic relationships. These are based on research findings, common experiences, and societal trends. But it should be acknowledged that every person and relationship is unique. And even when I cite statistics and scientific findings to illustrate a tendency, standard, or biological fact, there will still be exceptions.

The advice given in this book, therefore, should be taken as general guidance because it's not possible to cover all possible permutations and exceptions that may exist in individual relationships. What works for one may not work for another. I've made every effort to provide useful and relevant recommendations applicable to most situations. Please consider them all in the context of your own unique circumstances.

For the purposes of brevity and clarity, I have focused on cis-heterosexual men in a committed romantic relationship— those living with or not living with a partner, considering tying or who've recently tied the knot, or who are already deeply woven into the fabric of marriage. It could also be for those who have broken free of such ties but who are open to finding love again. Of course, the advice and principles discussed here could also be helpful to others. Anyone and everyone is welcome to read it and take what they believe could be applicable to their own issues of the heart.

As a focal point though, this book is dedicated to all the decent, peace-loving men who aim to protect and provide, honor, and cherish. (It's definitely not for those dealing with serious issues like misogyny, Intimate Partner Violence, and such. That's not something a mere book can address.) It's not going to give dating advice or how to make that great first impression so you're sure to get a second date and more. This is for those who've had their share of serial dating and situationships. It's for those in pursuit of real love and wanting to know what to look for. Or those who believe they've found it and want to make it last.

Many of the men who've picked up this book may feel happy being with their partner—and yet remain baffled because whatever they're doing now doesn't seem to be enough. Just as an example, my conflict avoidance in hopes of sidestepping irreparable damage ended up causing it instead. You may be wondering how a couple could go thirty years together without a single fight. We did have civil "discussions." That's to say, contained and restrained conversations that often left things unresolved because we both refused to engage in a battle of wills. But that doesn't mean allowing tempers to flare is the answer either. And it's not about simply "finding a balance." There's much, much more to keeping the peace than that; so to help with this, I've included a section on conflict management in chapter 5, under Rule No. 3.

Marriage, or any committed relationship, is a tango. Two people in a dance where things can flow smoothly until somebody steps on the other's toes or stumbles or decides to dance with somebody else. So, even as I tackle the topic of romantic relationships from a man's perspective, I'm well aware that it takes two to make it work.

That being said, I hope it's clear that I'm not putting the onus of having a good relationship on men and men alone. This book explores only one side of the equation. It's me, sharing my newfound perspective—a point of view any cis-heterosexual man can take when it comes to the art and skill of loving a woman.

Parts of this book will enlighten, surprise, and move you. Others will upset, disturb, or trigger you. It would be good to take note of those parts and how they made you feel because they could be hinting at things you value in life, or inner truths and hidden narratives that need to be explored. It's important to keep those in mind.

Who May Not Benefit Much from This Book

Yes, you may say, it's a given that it takes two to tango. What you may not have considered is that not everyone can tango. By that, I mean that there are certain personality types who are ill-equipped to have healthy, mutually beneficial relationships.

I'm talking about negative but non-pathological personality traits, initially identified as the dark triad, namely Machiavellianism, sub-clinical narcissism, and sub-clinical psychopathy. Dark triad is a term coined for a theory of personality first published in 2002 in the Journal of Research and Personality by psychologists Delroy Paulhus and Kevin

Williams. In 2019, other psychologists suggested expanding the concept to include sadism, forming a dark tetrad.

I will touch on this topic briefly because it could be of help to those who might have encountered such personalities within their families, work environment, or in their relationships—romantic or otherwise. Having this information could shed light on why maintaining relationships with such personality types will always be challenging, if not ill-advised.

The Dark Tetrad Personality Types

Machiavellianism, named after the Italian political philosophy of Niccolò Machiavelli, is marked by a tendency to be highly manipulative. People with this trait will deceive others to get what they want, have a cynical view of the world, and are good at deception.

Narcissism is a term derived from Greek mythology. Those familiar with it might mistake the trait as simply meaning being excessively concerned about one's appearance. Under this theory of personality, it goes much deeper than that. It's a trait marked by feelings of entitlement, dominance, a grandiose self-view, and attention-seeking. Narcissists can be hypersensitive to criticism, intolerant, and controlling so as to make everything going on around them to be about pleasing or serving them.

As for psychopathy, the key traits include callousness, impulsiveness, and being prone to taking big risks. It's an antisocial personality trait that makes it difficult for a psychopathic person to perceive and understand another's emotions due to a lack of empathy.

Everyday sadism is a negative personality type that finds pleasure in the suffering of others, simply defined as the enjoyment of cruelty. Although sadists often display physical aggression, it could also be manifested by trolling others on social media for the sheer fun of it.

A Chance at Long-Term Relationships?

Despite the "sinister" descriptions above, it can be challenging to recognize when someone has one or more of these traits. This is because they make a good first impression displaying extraverted behavior and are likely to be charming and charismatic. It's also difficult for psychologists to ascertain how many people fit within the dark tetrad description because, technically, these aren't official diagnoses found in the Diagnostic and Statistical Manual of Mental Disorders (the latest edition, the DSM-5-TR, was published in 2022). Based on available data, however, these negative personality traits are reasonably common, and they occur at subclinical levels, so people with these tendencies, in varying degrees, can blend in and live normal lives.

Studies consistently show that the dark tetrad traits are more prominent in men than in women. Not surprisingly, one study has shown that these personality traits correlate with frequent and more-hostile disagreements in romantic relationships.[1]

If, as you were reading the descriptions above, you recognized any of these traits in your partner or in yourself, then all the advice and insights in this book—and many other self-growth books combined—may not be enough to address your situation. Instinctively, you may resist the notion that you, or your partner, need any professional help. But if you are truly serious about finding stability and lasting calm in your long-term relationship, do reach out to a therapist or counselor. As I said at the start of this section, not all people can tango. There's a chance even these people can—with some professional guidance.

1

A Hero's Journey

Long before they're ready, young boys are told to "Be a man." They're told not to cry, to suck it up, and even with a bleeding wound on one knee, are told to go back to the playing field because they'll be all right. Boys grow up believing emotions should be shoved to the side or buried deep inside; then one day, they meet a woman whose mere presence challenges their vise-like grip on their feelings. And this feminine, nurturing, emotionally generous person speaks in a language alien to the masculine mind.

What you have in your hand is a guidebook on adult relationships that aims to pin down the elusive answer to the question "What does a woman want?"—and help men find some clarity.

This book is a journey that will help you understand her and relate to her better. But it begins with a look within *you* because half of any romantic relationship will always be made up of you. So if there's anything you can take full responsibility for, it's going to be your half.

According to a 2015 research study led by the American Sociological Association, nearly 70% of divorces are initiated by the wife. Among college-educated women, this number goes up to a staggering 90%.

Drawing on the research and science I've learned—and bringing that wisdom into sharper focus through the lens of my own experiences—I have identified three key rules that men can follow to help them navigate the complexities of love so they can cultivate peace, emotional intimacy, and happiness in their romantic relationships.

For those who want to cut to the chase, I'm stating the three rules right here:

1. Know Who You Love—and Why: The magnet that will pull you two together for the right reasons

2. Do Things that Show Her You Love Her: The unexpected aphrodisiac that redefines your definition of foreplay

3. Feel Your Feelings and Soften Them Up: The challenge to shed the armor and open your heart to vulnerability

Simply put, the rules are about recruiting three things into the quest of loving a woman: your mind, your actions, and your heart. That should make things incredibly easy to remember. It's deceptively basic and seemingly a no-brainer. But if it were really that easy, then why are so many relationships tangled up in knots?

The rest of this book will contain the detailed answers as to why you need these rules and how to go about applying them. We'll be going through some fundamental first steps that are crucial to understanding your state of mind as well as explanations and examples of the principles behind the rules. In going through this process, I've taken on the task of filling in a void in the lives of men and their romantic relationships: The absence of role models.

When it comes to loving a woman, men have no heroes. Most men, in fact, model their behavior from the example set by their fathers who were raised to be stone-faced gladiators. Soldiers of success. Warriors in the boardroom—and the bedroom.

You, holding this book, have evolved to the point of understanding that wanting to love—and wanting to know how to love—no longer holds the stigma it used to have. But much of the world still has some catching up to do, so that doesn't make things easy for most men.

Science provides data that proves men are biologically the more aggressive,[2] risk-taking,[3] lustier[4] sex— but at the same time, are in fact born more emotionally expressive than women.[5] Culturally, however, they are raised to keep their emotions tightly guarded; and they're supposed to avoid saying, doing, or displaying anything that could be interpreted as a sign of weakness. This combination of nature and nurture that molds men into emotionally unavailable individuals makes them seem like unsuitable recruits for an army of men out to conquer women's hearts through acts of love, thoughtfulness, and romance. But the good news is that men also have agency—the ability to act on one's own will or have independent control of one's actions.

This book will fortify that ability, by taking the most iconic heroes and superheroes—from olden times to the modern—then reappropriate them as role-models-with-a-twist for men in love today. I'll be recruiting them as guides as I take you through your own hero's journey. They'll be examples set to help men who falter, fumble, and eventually fall in love—so they can land solidly in a superhero pose. One hand and one knee placed squarely on the ground, and the other hand raised to the sky.

Read this book and join an army of Brave Hearts. Because it takes courage to enter a committed relationship—and faith to believe that it can last the challenges of time. The heart is fragile, and most people are afraid to break it. But we need to step forward and risk it.

Love can die. Unless we fight for it.

2

IN SEARCH OF HEROES

I READ SOMEWHERE THAT recruiting an all-volunteer military is a formidable task. Yet that's exactly what I'm doing. I am enlisting an army of men to pick up this book and, in reading it, join me on a trek across miles of self-discovery. It's basic training towards becoming part of the Brave Hearts Brigade.

We stand here, at the beginning of our journey with a vast landscape up ahead, with you standing on an outcrop and holding this guidebook in your hand. This book serves as a map for those who have a vague notion they're lost—even though it seems they know exactly where they are: They're with a woman whom they love.

Why does the man feel disoriented? He listens when she speaks, yet she still feels unheard. He takes her out whenever he has the chance, but she still feels neglected. He helps whenever she asks, gives her gifts he chose himself, and works his ass off in order to provide, yet she wonders if he still loves her.

"Where the hell am I?" The men wonder as they stare at this page.

The simple answer is that you're at the beginning of a quest. A hero's quest to find the answer to a puzzle that for a long time has remained unsolved. *What does a woman want?*

I'm in search of heroes, those who've been wounded and scarred, whether from past or on-going relationships, yet are still willing to bare their chest and expose their hearts. To open their minds to see things from her perspective. To perform acts that demonstrate his love in ways that matter to her.

In the end, you will be standing in the company of heroes at heart, in mind, and in their deeds.

Let's begin by taking a look at how this company of men started out in life.

A Look Back in Time

When I ask people, "What did love look like?"—they're almost always at a loss.

Perhaps the oddity of the question is why anyone would be caught off guard by it. But the more likely reason is because none of us really have a clear and authenticated idea of what romantic love in this decade really looks like.

There's a term in psychology called *modeling* which means learning by copying the behavior of someone else. It happens when a certain behavior is observed from a role model and the one who sees it learns that behavior and carries it on. For example, how a child learns to use a knife and fork is by copying grownups at the dining table. As a less obvious example, it's been suggested that most smokers pick up the habit after they see someone they look up to puffing on a cigarette, and they later on try it out themselves.

Similarly, the way we love is often a product of modeling. So it became my norm, as I started my practice as counselor, to always ask this question early on: What did love look like?

The image of love that lies in our subconscious was formed by the people we trusted most in our childhood. The couple who became the symbol of union in our innocent eyes. They showed us how a man and woman in a long-term relationship are supposed to treat one another.

What did love between your father and mother look like? Or if you were raised by a single parent or another caregiver, what do you remember of any interaction this person had with someone they loved romantically?

The answers I get for this question are wide-ranging. Anything from "a lot of fighting" to "they were just there" to "marriage was a duty" to "it was warm." The vast majority of answers are usually variations of the first two. If the way we love our long-term partners is highly influenced by modeling, and we were raised in a home where the open expression of romantic love was hardly present, then how can we demonstrate our love if we don't even know what it looks like?

Another question I ask is, "What did love look like between you and your mother (or primary caregiver)?" Think back to when you were a child, and I don't mean when you were sixteen, thirteen, or ten. I mean further back in time—as close as you can bring yourself to being a preschooler. Of course, the phenomenon of childhood amnesia makes us forget what life was like before we were four years of age. But try closing your eyes and concentrate, then allow yourself to bring up memories of your mother or other primary caregiver as far back in time as you can. Maybe you were somewhere between five and seven at the time.

Was your primary caregiver (this could be either of your parents or a guardian) demanding and controlling? Or, let's say your primary caregiver was your mother—was she always too busy to take care of your needs? Or maybe she was the opposite and relied heavily on you because your father wasn't around. If you came to her in pain or in need of comfort, did she offer you another feeling with which to substitute your distress? Or perhaps your primary caregiver was your father? Were you shamed or shunned for asking to be comforted? Did he often say, "Don't worry about it. You'll be fine." Or was your most trusted caregiver responsive to your needs. Did he or she ask what you were feeling and take the time to help you sort through your troubles?

Our emotional responsiveness is often modeled after how others had responded to our feelings when we were children. This isn't to lay any blame on our parents or caregivers. They were dealing with life and love the best way they knew how—which was also modeled after their own parents.

It travels through generations, this ignorance of ours as to what good love looks like. When asked to paint a picture of it in the present age, we often turn to what movies and novels and love songs tell us. In other words, our modified picture of romantic love—how we believe it ought to look like—is often based on fiction.

When it comes to romantic love, therefore, most of us have no real-world examples of men who've been doing it the right way. A man's father, brothers, uncles, workmates, teammates, and drinking buddies are seldom, if ever, considered authorities when it comes to loving a woman in ways that leave both husband and wife happy. There were exceptions, of course, but men generally end up challenged by an idealistic picture painted by chick flicks, romance novels, and sentimental lyrics—and men believe it's a picture that's meant for women to fantasize about but impossible for men to live up to.

Perhaps hoping for a woman who will be perfectly happy and absolutely devoid of complaints is a picture for men to fantasize about and one which is impossible to obtain. Yet the rules I'll be presenting, at the very least, will help give men some simple things they can apply immediately and bring them closer to the achievable ideal relationship every couple hopes for.

In the Company of Other Men

Having had no "drill sergeants" to train them on how to engage with the other party on the rough terrain of love and romantic relationships, most men choose to make up their own strategies when they land in that alien territory. They go by what's familiar to them from childhood, or by avoiding what got them stunned and wounded in previous relationships, plus some pointers and tricks they picked up from other soldiers marching down the same trail.

Generally, men end up falling under one of four "armored units" each with its own set of tactics on how to win in this "heart-to-heart combat." I call these units The Brave Hearts Brigade, The Dodger Division, The Saintly Squadron, and The Pondering Platoon.

The Brave Hearts Brigade

A man who is now in a satisfying and happy long-term relationship is someone I'd say is already in the Brave Hearts unit. Being brave-hearted, he's put away his hostility, laid down his weapons and shield, and opened up his heart to the woman he loves. Allowing himself to be vulnerable, he'll be living life and loving his significant other with the kindness, respect, and whole-hearted supportiveness this book prescribes. Quite likely, he grew up in a secure environment with emotionally available caregivers, equipping him with the sense of wholeness needed to face the challenges of a romantic relationship. If his life's path had led him to a woman with the same emotional maturity and whose values are compatible with his, then he's now blessed with a warm and loving relationship he'd grown up knowing was possible. It still has its struggles, but since they both understand what brings peace into their union, they deal with their problems together and not against each other.

It's also possible he used to fight for love in one of the other units and has since learned what it truly takes to win as half of a couple, eventually becoming one of the Brave Hearts.

The Dodger Division

Those who signed up to this unit look perfectly in control of their lives. And no wonder! They were most likely raised in an environment that required them to become independent and look after themselves. They work hard and play hard. They probably go out of their way to help others; they also help with the household chores and are good fathers and good providers. What isn't apparent to most people, including the man himself, is that all these activities now serve as ways of dodging getting emotionally intimate with his partner. All the late nights at work, the side hustles, the time spent at the gym, with his parents, his kids, his pets, his buddies, his car, his booze, his hobbies (and maybe even a mistress) are all there to keep him from spending time that would require him to be vulnerable with his wife. He'd rather occupy his time with everything else—even if it's just porn, a rerun of a game, scrolling through social media, or even faking a dire need for sleep—rather than talk to the woman living under the same roof about how tired and frustrated and lonely he feels in their relationship.

These men believe they are living a well-rounded life, and it may seem so too. But the hidden catch about how those in the Dodger Division face the other camp is to simply block and sabotage any chance of free time being dedicated to emotional vulnerability with his partner.

The Saintly Squadron

Maybe you can guess from the name of this unit that its recruits are men who seem to deserve a halo for openly demonstrating their devotion to their wives or girlfriends. They are also good providers who help a lot around the house, doing most, if not all, of the chores. Then even though they're tired from work, they spend time listening to their partner's stories and grievances about her day. When they're with family and friends, they're extra attentive to their wife, getting the food and drinks for her, accompanying her if she needs to go anywhere, constantly asking if she needs anything. Always demonstrating how he's the perfect gentleman to his partner, he would loudly declare how beautiful, smart, and sexy she is, or maybe crack jokes about how afraid he is of losing her or that her wish is his command. He'd even post about his adulation of his partner on social media. Men in the Saintly Squadron may also be called the Good Boys. The Nice Guys. Maybe even Mama's Boys. The ones who were properly trained by their mothers on how to treat a woman right.

Unfortunately, this training usually involved the suppression of their own desires and feelings. Quite the opposite of those in the Dodger Division who were primed to depend on themselves, the Saintly Squadron grew up feeling their caregivers depended on them a lot. They may have suffered emotional neglect or enmeshment in their early years and learned to serve women because that was how they believed they could get love in return. In looking after his caregiver's needs (e.g. an alcoholic father, a mentally unstable mother), he manufactured some form of attention. But now that he's a grown man, sticking to this childhood dynamic confuses him when, no matter how much he gives or no matter how hard he tries, his partner remains unsatisfied and unavailable for sex. She always has something to correct about what he did, some other errand or task for him to do, or one more thing she wants him to buy. But he takes the complaints and criticism then goes ahead and does the added chores and buys that new item she asked for without so much as a grimace. Deep inside, he may be thinking that once he gets things right and her list of things-to-do gets accomplished, he'll get the happy relationship he's been hoping for. He's heard it said so many times before: Happy wife, happy life. And he believes it. Except he has no idea when she'd be happy. And so he keeps up the saintly act, rather than talk to her about his sadness, frustrations, and unmet needs.

The Pondering Platoon

The Pondering Platoon is composed of men who often find themselves puzzled as they stand guard over their boundaries. They aim to be flexible. They want to be able to be give more without losing too much of themselves. But they ended up with someone whose needs they couldn't fully comprehend, and now, they're faced with that problem.

Unlike those in the Dodger Division who excessively fill up their calendars, the Pondering Platoon strives for a balance between freedom and couple-dom. Similar to those in the Saintly Squadron, a man in this unit also demonstrates his devotion and respect for his partner, helping and supporting her as best he can, while ensuring that his personal time and space are respected too.

For someone in the Pondering Platoon, caring for someone often feels like a conundrum he needs to crack. He ends up studying the relationship, trying to solve the issues through a push-and-pull struggle over boundaries. He finds himself overthinking, as though figuring out a Rubik's cube one twist and turn at a time. Or strategizing, ready for a game of Minesweeper. And for a variety of reasons, all this puzzle-solving could remain stalled. Perhaps he ended up with someone who couldn't understand the extent of his boundaries. Or he could be battling an adversary who has no control over her hurricane of feelings. It's also possible he's in a relationship with a female member of the Dodger Division, and she's the one who immerses herself in work, motherhood, homemaker duties, and other pursuits, keeping herself cold and distant despite his desire for warmth and closeness. Faced with either a woman who weeps through every conflict, or one who doesn't fight fair and uses painful tactics that demean, attack, and insult his pride, or another one who considers him as just one more thing she needs to pencil into her calendar, a guy in the Pondering Platoon may be at a loss on how to win the battle. So he keeps his true feelings to himself and builds walls around him instead, keeping his loneliness and frustration locked inside a fortress until he figures out what to do.

Where to From Here

We've glanced behind us to have a look at childhood memories and see the beginnings of how men learned to deal with their daily battles. Then we paused at the start of our hero's journey to check out which of the "armed units" men might find themselves in.

As you can probably tell, it's possible for one man to have been in each of the units at one time or another. The common thread between the Dodger Division, Saintly Squadron, and Pondering Platoon is that they're all unable or unwilling to express their sentiments regarding how their partner is engaging with them—even when it's pushed them into a hidden depression. (There are also men who just don't sign up to any kind of company and go by their own rules. Usually, these are men with the dark personality traits we discussed in the preface. They aren't team players and will have a difficult time maintaining meaningful relationships without counseling.)

I have simplified the Brave Hearts guidebook as best as I could, despite modern love and romantic relationships proving to be a difficult territory to navigate. But the reason it's difficult is because men and women grew up without being taught and properly guided on how to go about it right. And because of our ignorance, it has turned success in romantic relationships into a guessing game.

As we progress on this journey, we'll be filling up what we'll call a "Knapsack of Knowledge." It's bound to get heavier as we move along, so it will be good to take an inventory now and then to make sure we're not forgetting anything.

To keep things simple, I've clustered my findings and insights about men and relationships under three pillars or rules. Under these, I'll associate the ideas with iconic male figures to help crystallize what the three rules mean as portrayed—or not—by these heroes, old and new.

Men need heroes. And for the most part, they have role models, idols, or icons—many of them unreal or surreal or semi-real (like celebrities and their public personas)—who become part of their hodge-podge definition of what makes a man ... a "man." I went in search of heroes who could serve as role models for men on how to love a woman in terms that even women would agree with, but it seems that no famous man is held in such high regard by the world. In fact, women have no generally-accepted role model either, because unlike our careers and public life, our romantic lives are mostly kept secret. Being successful in love and marriage has also had ever evolving standards. There was a time when love wasn't even considered necessary for marriage at all.

There are, for certain, real-life role models, and as a result of my declaration of being unable to find them, I hope people will start sharing their stories so that others may learn. For now, let's go with iconic fictional characters that I will be using as examples for different ingredients to modern love.

Let's take the first step into our quest that involves finding the seeds of the hero that lies within ourselves.

3

Rule No. 1: Know Who You Love — and Why

"What does a woman want?" It's a question Sigmund Freud had declared he'd failed to answer, despite his thirty years of research into what he called "the feminine soul."

It's a question that continues to baffle men to this day. Somewhere in the middle of this book, I've buried my answer to that question, much like hidden treasure. Everything from here to there is like a map you and I will need to follow, so our thoughts don't get lost along the way.

Meanwhile, allow me to take you back in time—much, much farther back than the mere three decades in which Freud conducted his research. Let's rewind to one pre-historic day for a quick glimpse at how the minds of men and women grew to be so different from one another.

Meet Brongk. He's a cave boy who's been brought along by his father for his first hunt with two other men of the tribe. They've been walking all day, it's late afternoon, and Brongk's stomach is grumbling.

"I'm hungry," he tells his father, scratching an itch near his groin underneath the animal hide his mother had told him to wear for this trek.

His father, Drrahd grunts, tears off some jerky from the stash in his pouch, and hands it to the boy.

Brongk bites into the dry and tough meat, wondering if it could taste better. He wishes he were back home, eating the sweet, juicy fruit and crunchy nuts his mother would have handed him. He also wishes he could learn how to cure meat better instead of being one of the hunters walking in the heat.

"I miss Mom," Brongk says.

Drrahd turns to him, his thick brows scrunched, then conks him on the head. "You idiot. We're hunting mammoths. We could get attacked by wolves, and you're thinking of your mama? What are you, a baby?"

The other men laugh. One crumples up his face and pretends to wail like an infant. The other laughs louder. Brongk winces inwardly, looks up at his father, and fears he has let the big man down.

"Keep your mind on the hunt." His father growls. "Our lives depend on each other while we're out here. You cannot be weak. The tribe depends on our success. They depend on our strength."

An image of the tribe rejoicing at their return with their haul of fresh meat flashes in Brongk's mind. The larger the game they bring home, the higher they will be regarded. He pictures the joy and relief on his mother's face at the sight of him and his father returning safe and unharmed.

Brongk understands with more clarity the importance of his job. It's bigger than a mammoth. Others of the tribe will teach him about spears and knives. How to make, sharpen, and use them to provide precious meat, kill predators, and to protect their tribe from men of other tribes. He will be taught strategy, skill, endurance, and courage. Nothing else must disturb his mind while he's focused on the job. His job is the purpose of his life.

Meanwhile, back at the caves, his mother, Kro-ah, is rushing back to the caves with the other tribeswomen who've been out gathering nuts and fruits with her. Though their main task is to find food, Kro-ah has a mental list of other things she's been ticking off. She's found some yarrow, lemon balm, and purple betony that the herbalist has asked her to keep an eye out for. She's also gathered some vines for new baskets her elder cousin needed to make. The other women have their own things to collect. Stones, sticks, and tree sap. Bugs, bones, and tree bark. The women keep up a chatter, reminding each other of the different things everyone back home might need. This is prehistoric times, you see, so the idea of simply heading out with a list in hand is beyond them. They have no word for "family" yet either. Everyone is looking out for everyone's kin, so their concerns encompass the entire tribe.

Which is why they're hurrying back—hurrying yet still pausing now and then because someone spotted or remembered something for somebody. It's because a friend's grandma could barely see, a neighbor's uncle has a broken leg, another's sister could give birth any minute, and a cousin's baby has a fever.

There are many other things on their communal mental list of cares. All of these are Kro-ah's concerns too because all the women need each other to hold it all together. They have become the "rememberers" of the tribe. While the men are away, they have to make sure everyone gets food at particular times of the day; that the caves and all clothing are cleaned, babies are breastfed, tears are dried, upset stomachs, lice-infested heads, fresh and healing wounds are tended to, baskets and pelts are mended and made, no one dies from illness or childbirth, falls from a tree, gets blinded in a stick fight, singed by fire, stung by a bee, or wanders off into the woods and gets attacked by a wild animal. It's a blessing that the children have no homework and soccer practice in this era.

Thunder rumbles overhead, and Kro-ah's mind instantly centers on one concern as her heart throbs for her eldest son, Brongk, who is out on his first hunt. Then her thoughts fly to Brongk's father, Drrahd. He's a bold man; she fears he will one day die from his bravery. She sends out a prayer to the souls of the departed. *Please look after them and keep them safe.*

The women around her notice her tense up, and her mother, standing by her, caresses her arm.

"Brongk will be all right," Mom says. "He's a strong boy."

The others smile and add their reassurances. A few of them start telling tales of their own worries when their sons went out on their first hunts too.

Kro-ah listens and accepts their outpouring of support, grateful that she has a tribe to help her raise her son—and look after everyone else's children, and their elders, their tribesmen, and each other. Many of these women are also good hunters, just like Kro-ah and her mother. But the hunting grounds for big game are far away, so they chose to forage close by for the little children—in fact, for the entire tribe who depend on the women for every mealtime. It's a lesson she's been learning every day of her life. Her concerns are bigger than herself. Nothing and no one can be forgotten. Everyone and everything related to the well-being of the tribe is her job.

I won't claim that this is pre-historically accurate down to every detail. But largely, it can hold up to evolutionary scrutiny. Recent archeological findings[6] prove that a majority of pre-historic women were also hunters. And for societies that subsisted on foraging and hunting, the men's contribution to the food supply was largely through the hunt. The foragers were almost always women.

It was an early human world that thrived with men as highly-focused hunters and women as multitasking gatherers. It's a contrast that made their partnership work well when the world was how it was. The women supported the men's hyperfocus and steeliness, and the men appreciated the women's ultrawide scope of attention and worrying ways.

It's a difference molded by our beginnings as a race. The human race. The male and female brains evolved differently for the survival of the species. Research suggests that male-female brain differences[7] may be genetically hard-wired even before the flood of testosterone and estrogen that happens during fetal development which further delineates those differences. One's upbringing, society, and culture, thereafter, step in and continue to sculpt the male or female that emerges.

Boys were raised to lay down their lives for the tribe and face danger without fear. Girls were raised to take care of the tribe and always fear for everyone's safety.

Modern-day Hunters and Gatherers

Today, the world has completely transformed, and we're stymied and stunned by each other's peculiar attitudes and behaviors. There have been monumental shifts in the roles men and women fulfill, while the stereotypes from long ago prevail but have lost much of their significance. Men are still pressured to be serious hunters focused on bringing home the big game and women are branded as nit-picking talkative "rememberers." It's no wonder modern men and women, even when in love, can end up getting on each other's nerves.

Men and women have become strangers to one another. But the worst part is, after a boy is told to shut out his feelings, ignore his thoughts about the motherly care that he's missing, turn his back on the things he'd rather do instead of what his tribe expects him to do, he becomes a stranger to himself.

Rule No. 1 is a two-pronged rule. It's about knowing the woman you love—and understanding why you do. Answering that second part requires some self-awareness.

So before I usher you deeper into these pages, let me ask you a few questions to see how well you know yourself. You've spent most of your life ignoring, denying, and covering up your feelings. Now that you're in a relationship, contemplating, or healing from one—how do you know what's real about what you feel?

Are you really in love? Or are you simply in a relationship? Or do you just need to be in one, so you're not the guy without a girl?

Many people end up in relationships, or stay in one, for reasons far removed from love. The push could easily come from hormones, the desire to have kids, societal and peer pressure, or sheer loneliness. That's why the first of the three rules to love and live by is about getting your mind in on the act of loving.

The key to a healthy, romantic relationship is to know yourself. A deep level of self-awareness and self-acceptance. Only then can a man move on to find the woman who can love that man who he has defined—and continues to refine—as the self he can be proud of.

If, after some soul searching, you come to realize that you mistook her looks and your lust for love, or that you got drawn in when she chased you and made a relationship seem easy, or you settled for the safer choice, that person who will never hurt or leave you—then you may want to turn what you have into something deeper. One other thing that could happen as you read on is that you'll come to a crossroads and need to decide if life is too short to be with the wrong person.

Let me start by re-introducing you to some heroes who can help men see love from new perspectives and gain a new vision for themselves. Let's begin this journey of becoming a braver heart by having a look inside you.

BE ETHAN HUNT. KNOW YOUR MISSION. IT'S NOT IMPOSSIBLE.

RULE NO. 1: KNOW WHO YOU LOVE—AND WHY

The road ahead is full of twists and turns and the iconic character who's going to lead us into Rule No. 1 is Ethan Hunt, a highly skilled operative of the Impossible Mission Force. An agent of true grit, Ethan flashes us a smile, exuding the confidence that helps him tackle every *Mission: Impossible.*

He starts by handing each of us a compass to clip on our camo knapsacks. He's wearing dark glasses, but you can still feel his piercing gaze on you when he deposits a compass in your hand. "Are you ready?"

You clear your throat and ask, "Uhm ... for what?"

"We're here to find your mission." He checks his own compass then nods in the direction we're supposed to take. He marches off towards it, leading us down the path of Rule No. 1.

He's going at a fast pace, so you call out after him, "We need to find it?" You scratch your head. "Don't they just give it to you, and you get to choose to accept it or not?"

Ethan stops dead in his tracks, stands stock still, then slowly pivots to face you. "Your mission," he says through gritted teeth, "should you choose to accept it, is to find out what it is."

You hold your mouth agape for a moment. "Say what?"

"This is all about you," Ethan says. "It's not for anyone to tell you what it is." He takes off his sunglasses, looks you straight in the eye, and asks, "Are you committed to seeing this through until the goal is accomplished?"

You swallow and nod hesitantly.

He smiles then slips his sunglasses back on. "Let's go."

We rush to follow him down this road of self-discovery.

Before any man sets his sights on any woman for "the kill," he needs to have a dossier on himself. He needs to ask himself: *What is my mission in life?* Every individual who desires a relationship has a purpose outside of that relationship. No person is limited to just being a husband or wife or a committed partner—well, at least, they shouldn't be. Multiple research studies have shown how leading a meaningful life contributes to one's physical health, mental fitness, and longevity.

Ideally, one's partner becomes one's companion and supporter as we go about fulfilling our purpose in life. When each half of a couple respects and believes in the other's mission, it gives that relationship much greater chances of staying healthy, happy, and growing stronger through the years. When visions and expectations collide, rifts can form and create distance between two people.

So now, on this hero's journey, Ethan Hunt challenges us with a goal: to find out your own personal mission. It's your turn to find what matters most to you, so you can nurture a relationship with a woman who supports that mission. In other words, through this exercise, you'll be on your way to *Mission: Compatible.*

To know your purpose, you need to know your inner self and understand your needs, strengths, and core values. If a man lacks self-awareness and falls short of accepting himself in any of the key pillars of self-growth, he could be using relationships as a crutch or as a means to love the parts of himself he can't love.

In this section, let's put together your dossier to guide you in identifying your mission. All you need to do is take three simple steps:

STEP ONE: Take control of your life.

STEP TWO: Take stock of your core values.

STEP THREE: Take charge of a change in the world.

Let's take these one step at a time.

STEP ONE: Take Control of Your Life

There are many aspects to a person's life that, all in all, help define him. They're like pillars that hold up his perception of his self-worth. To take control, the key is to assess your situation in each of these pillars—so you get to see your triumphs and your tribulations with more clarity.

"Why do we need to go through this?" you ask, glancing at me.

"Because you need to be sure you're not looking for issues or solutions *outside* of you," I say, "to address pain points that can only be resolved from *inside* of you."

You shake your head. "I don't get it."

Ethan steps forward to stand between you and me. "Two words," he says, holding up two fingers in a V.

"Mission impossible?" you guess.

"Conflict resolution," Ethan says.

You squint at him. "Isn't that the same thing?" You let out a snort. "I mean, there's just no getting rid of conflict, right?"

"Right," Ethan says. "But you." He jabs a finger into your chest. "You need to be honest with yourself. Take a long hard look inside for things you're hiding. Denying. Disguising. Old beliefs you're guarding for reasons you don't even know. A lot of times, that's where conflict starts."

Ethan is talking about the chance of you thinking that the whole issue is only your relationship when maybe it isn't. Insecurities. Fears. Traumas. This exercise will point towards any inner work that needs to be done so the burden of dealing with these issues won't fall on your partner's shoulders, because it's not her job to fix you. She can support and understand you, but the "cleaning up" starts from within.

This part of the hero's journey brings us to the gates of a huge house. We'll be staying here for a while as we go inside and look around the different rooms. This "house" is actually a metaphor for you. You can imagine it however you wish, to be reflective of yourself, inside and out.

Ethan unlocks the gates and swings them open. We walk up to the front door, and he instructs us to have a tour of the place. We need to check out which rooms will make you proud when visitors get to see them, which ones need a bit of dusting, and which might be in sort of a mess and will need some work.

As we go through each one, ask yourself, is your current state "Really Good?" "Just Fine?" Or "Pretty Bad?"

1.Social state: This is about your relationships with family and friends and their profound effect on everything else.

Back in 1938, Harvard researchers began a study to find out: What is the key to a happy life? Many people might assume it's fame or fortune.

Others might think it's the opposite, such as a spiritual life of simple pleasures. Eighty-five years later, Harvard reiterates the findings of the longest study ever conducted on happiness.[8] The key to joy, it revealed, is good relationships. Simply put, people who spent more positive time with others reported more feelings of happiness.

We're social creatures. We're wired to enjoy being in the company of others, whether family or friends. But there are also research studies that expose a sad reality among men. A 2021 survey[9] found that only 27% of men have six or more close friends, while 28% of men under the age of 30 reported having no close social connections at all.

The world of men is a hostile, competitive, and combative place. Even among the best of buddies, you can be attacked for simply showing up with product in your hair or for growing bald; shamed for not having a girlfriend or for letting on that you have feelings for a girl; jeered at for looking like a loser in a beat-up car or making up for a small dick with a sports coupe. And what's expected is that you grin or laugh through it all. These attacks to your pride and self-esteem are all part of the brotherhood. To keep you strong and safe from becoming, God forbid, anything like a girl.

Men cluster their friends based on shared activities, which is generally where their conversations revolve—shared interests and passions that don't have much to do with those inner facets of themselves. His work buddies know him differently from his soccer buddies; who'd be different still from his drinking buddies. If he's religious, he'd have a different group of brothers from church.

For women, friends are friends alike. All of them get the privilege of pouring their hearts out and baring their souls to one another—often with no need for social lubricants.

Many men report that most of their social bonding time happens in the context of alcohol consumption. According to research in *Clinical Psychological Science*, a journal of the Association for Psychological Science, alcohol is likely to induce some kind of "social bravery" among men, allowing them to be more responsive to another person's smile. This effect of having an increase in "contagious" smiles from alcohol was only seen in all-male groups—heterosexual men, in particular—suggesting that the alcohol disrupts some mental process that would normally prevent a man from responding to such gestures.

True and deep friendships among men may be as rare as 24k gold. Why? "Because they are men," says Professor Robin Dunbar, an anthropologist and evolutionary psychologist.[10]

This clash in research results—of close relationships being key to one's happiness versus the difficulty of men to forge deep friendships—gives us a clue as to why men tend to report higher levels of loneliness than women. According to a 2021 survey by the *Survey Center on American Life,* only 21% of men say they received emotional support from a friend within the past week, compared to 41% of women.

There's a silent epidemic of loneliness among men. My hope is that you have enough good relationships with family and friends to keep you from catching that loneliness bug.

So how are you when it comes to your social pillar?
A) Really Good   B) Just Fine   C) Pretty Bad

If you answered A, good for you! There's nothing more for you to do than keep enjoying it. Keep sharing the company of others. If you answered B or C, it would be good to assess who in your social circle supports you the most. List down the top three to five people who contribute to your goals and well-being. On the opposite end, enumerate those who drain you of your positivity. Those who weigh you down or discourage you.

Take control by increasing the time you spend with the uplifting people, and if possible, limit your exposure or even detach yourself altogether from those who pull you down. If you lack positive relationships in general, then find opportunities to make new friends or reconnect with those you may have drifted apart from. Start a hobby or a sport that's done in groups. Volunteer. Accept more invitations and attend social gatherings, even if it feels uncomfortable at first. Widening your circle needs to begin somewhere.

2.Physical state: Back in second grade, I was standing in line on the first day of school and my homeroom teacher caught sight of my tiny, scrawny frame, walked over to me, then said I didn't belong in her class. I gawped at her. I knew very well I was in the right class, but I just stood there in shock. She asked for my name and walked away. Instead of me thinking that she'd simply made a mistake and would figure this out after checking the class list, the only thought that emblazoned itself in my mind was that she found me so ugly, she wanted me out of her class at first sight. Minutes later, she returned and corrected herself, saying I did belong in her class. By that time, I was sobbing but I have no memory of whether she ever apologized. The damage had been done. She'd scarred me for life. Up until high school, every time I looked at my photographs, I saw a lizard staring back at me. I'm not kidding. My mind only saw what my second-grade homeroom teacher probably saw, a long, thin, pale face with droopy eyes devoid of any expression.

More than half a century has gone by since that day, but I still have doubts whenever someone says anything flattering or compliments how I look. Even though I was an ugly duckling who, I'd like to think, grew up to resemble something close to a swan, that "rejection-at-first-sight" moment never left me. That was a fleeting moment back in early grade school, but it shaped me. It's made me very conscientious about my overall health and how I groom myself, taking good care of my physique, posture, and my hair and skin (I fought hard to skip the severe acne stage my siblings went through in their teenage years).

Fast forward to me as a young university graduate in my first job in an ad agency. I was a junior copywriter in my early twenties, still pale and scrawny, armed with a bachelor's degree but with an overall countenance of someone still in high school. In client meetings, after I'd done my best to make a well-rehearsed, professional-caliber presentation of my advertising work, the first question the clients would invariably ask was, "How old are you?" A co-worker advised me to fix things by somehow adding some years to how I looked. So I enrolled in a gym to pad on a few pounds. Got a smart haircut and bought myself half a closet of clothes that said "corporate." My clients' comments, thereafter, pertained to my strategic thinking and creative work.

Fast forward even further to me in my early 40s, when I walked into a marketing event in jeans, leisure shoes, and a black T-shirt then headed for the buffet. A twenty-something junior marketing executive whom I'd briefly interacted with in a couple of meetings came up to me and said ... something that I found incoherent.

"Excuse me?" I asked.

I had to glance at the junior executive's lips to make sure the words coming out were what I thought I'd heard the first time. "You're so hot," came the exact same words.

"Oh," I said with a chuckle and wondered what had possessed the person. I don't remember if I even had the presence of mind to say thanks for the compliment, but I do know I quickly moved back to the buffet table to put something on my plate to avoid having to say anything more.

Good thing I'd taken care of my physical state even in my youth. It got me from being a scrawny lizard that a teacher had rejected to being the "hot" president and CEO of my own advertising agency.

All right, I admit, it's not exactly the gym membership, haircut, and clothes that got me where I am today. But these anecdotes serve to highlight my point. There are probably things you believe about yourself that are untruths put there by cruel things people said or did to you in your youth. They've turned into voices in your head, saying awful things full of doubt and negativity playing on repeat. Beyond that, there may also be real weaknesses you still have but are within your capacity to change—such as how you care for your body and how you present yourself physically to others. This pillar covers everything related to your overall physical state, such as your health, exercise, nutrition, sleep, hygiene, and looks.

How are you when it comes to your physical pillar?
A) Really Good   B) Just Fine   C) Pretty Bad

If you answered A, that's an awesome state to be in! If you chose B or C, aim for change and learn how to do better. If it concerns your health, consult a doctor. Diet, hygiene, and exercise are at your command. If you're overworking, over-exercising, getting high, drinking, overeating, starving yourself, not sleeping enough, or looking sloppy because you're not facing your feelings, reach out and talk with someone. Don't let your body and how you present yourself pay the price for problems your mind couldn't handle.

But what about a physical state that can't be changed by any amount of self-control, study, and deep conversations? What if you feel held back because of it? It's important to rise above this state of mind because it could lead a man towards self-sabotaging behavior when it comes to relationships, such that he might even question why a certain woman would stay faithful to him. It might even reach the point that he'd reject her—to beat her to the punch of rejecting him.

One's looks may be a major factor in triggering physical attraction. But that's not what counts the most for long-term relationships. In the 2019 Clue Ideal Partner Survey of 68,000 people from 180 countries, *kindness* was cited by nearly 90% of women as their most desirable trait in a partner. The other top traits selected by the women were *supportiveness* and *intelligence*, chosen by 86.5% and 72.3%, respectively. When it comes to physical traits, only 22.3% of women said an *attractive body* was very important, citing an *attractive smile* as the most important physical feature.

If you believe your ideal physical state is beyond attainment, then work towards gaining self-acceptance. Let's say, you're shorter than the average person and wished you were taller. You can boost your height a little with the right posture and shoes, and with sharper outfits, you could easily cut a fine figure. It's your aura of confidence that will make you ten feet tall.

But if your ideal is far beyond what is achievable, then practice self-compassion and offer yourself kindness too. Silence your inner critic and be forgiving of the things you can't change. A lot of times, we're harsher on ourselves than others are.

Pay attention to the positive relationships in your social circle. Embrace the company and camaraderie of people who accept, appreciate, and love you for all that you are. Much of the world has gone blind to many of the physical traits that used to divide us through discrimination. Look for role models out there who've achieved a great deal with the same physical traits you possess. If you can't find anyone, then it's your chance to become somebody's role model someday.

Take control through study, discipline, and self-acceptance. For those things that you can't physically change to the extent that you wish, you'll need to change your internal narrative. Connect more with people who like, support, and respect you. See who they see. And through their eyes, gain self-acceptance and self-love.

This acceptance needs to come from you—*first* of all and *above* all. It wouldn't be fair to your partner—perhaps a truly beautiful woman you're proud to have and to hold—if her main purpose is to bolster or be the provider of the confidence you couldn't find within yourself.

3.Marital state: The standard list of self-growth and wellness pillars normally doesn't include this, but I added it because it's a pain point for many people. I realize my choice of a term to identify this pillar could seem controversial or limiting to some. Many people these days no longer consider marriage the "end goal." The reason I elected to use the word *marital* is because it is still widely recognized as the legal term to identify one's status as either single, married, widowed, divorced, separated and, we can include, in a committed relationship of some kind other than married.

There are those who believe a romantic relationship is essential to happiness and satisfaction, while others find life more enjoyable and fulfilling without a partner. Elyakim Kislev, author of the book *Happy Singlehood* says long-term singles "cherish freedom, independence, and even creativity and nonconformity more than others." So a man may have chosen to get married because his experiences become richer with his wife by his side. Or someone could be single, happy, and in love but is worried about having to schedule his life around somebody else if he commits.

Included under your assessment of your marital state will also be your satisfaction with your sexual life. One can be single and highly active in dating apps or is content with time alone, a bottle of lotion, and a pack of Kleenex. Or one could be married and secure in his relationship but isn't getting enough sex.

I had initially subsumed the topic of sexual gratification under the previous pillar, meaning your physical state, because it's a biological need. Whether your sexual activity is with a partner or through masturbation, it's been proven to benefit your physical and mental health. But I decided to move sexuality under the marital pillar because whenever I ask someone to assess their physical well-being, they usually associate that with their physical appearance, overall health, diet, and exercise.

It's usually during discussions of marital contentment when the topic of unmet sexual needs comes up. Single men might have easy access to sexual partners but still feel "lacking." I've also had men declare profound love and respect for their wives but still find themselves looking outside the marriage for sexual gratification because he couldn't bring himself to face a difficult conversation about his sexual needs with his wife.

Sometimes, that yearning to get more—or better—could be the sole cause of why he feels wanting in his current marital state. Whether you're single or partnered up, giving yourself sexual satisfaction is good for your well-being. And sometimes, that could mean masturbation—the safest way to have sexual pleasure because it eliminates the risk of pregnancy, getting STIs, or falling in love with someone you barely know or shouldn't even be with.

[A side note on this topic: Make sure to practice healthy masturbation, keeping your attunement to your body and the sensations you experience as the source of pleasure —rather than being overly dependent on porn that might dampen your satisfaction once you're doing "the real thing" with a partner. Too much porn could lead to unrealistic expectations or create insecurities if you end up comparing yourself to unobtainable standards. Research has shown that exposure to porn makes people more critical of their partner's looks and rate themselves as less in love with their partner compared to those who didn't consume porn. Let me put it this way, if you get used to getting off only on roller coasters with loop-the-loops and turbo boosts, it's going to be tough enjoying the ride when the most that normal life can give you is being on cruise control in a nice sedan.]

I hope it's clear that in no way am I saying that you need to be married or in a romantic relationship to rate yourself as having a really good marital state. To quote Paul Tillich, "Our language has wisely sensed these two sides of man's being alone. It has created the word *loneliness* to express the pain of being alone. And it has created the word *solitude* to express the glory of being alone."

According to the data analysis done by the Pew Research Center of a 2019 census, about 38% of American adults ages 25 to 54 were unpartnered—meaning, neither married nor living with a partner. Quite a jump from 29% in 1990. Also, compared to thirty years ago, men are now more likely than women to be unpartnered. So, if you're single or married and happy the way things are, then assess your marital state as being really good. If you're a widower and still grieving but taking comfort in your memories, then you could say your state is just fine. If you're divorced, lonely, and still angry, then you might say you're in a pretty bad state for now.

So how are you when it comes to your marital pillar? How do you feel about it?

A) Really Good   B) Just Fine   C) Pretty Bad

If you answered A, I'm happy for you! If you answered B or C, I hope this checklist of pillars, as well as the rest of this book, will give you clarity on why you feel that way. Your loneliness might be stemming from some other pillar in your life, and finding out what it is will help you address it. You could be searching for something or someone in your life and not know what or who it is. Assessing yourself in the other pillars will help you get to know yourself better, and it might reveal that your "missing piece" is not related to your marital state at all but could be more about your social or recreational states or any of the others.

If you're single not by choice, being able to self-soothe in a healthy fashion can help keep you from rushing into a relationship if you aren't ready for one. Is a partner really what you need at this point in your life? Or is there first a hurdle you need to get past before you can   make any romantic relationship work—perhaps that of feeling whole and comfortable on your own.

Self-love will be discussed in more depth later in this section because enjoying your own company is crucial to being at ease with sharing yourself with a significant other. It can get really sad for a man to go on a never-ending search for a woman he could love when most of his thoughts about himself are negative. A romantic relationship isn't a cure for a lack of self-love. It won't be a true romance unless it's between two individuals who have accepted and embraced their own selves, imperfections and all. I'd like to underscore this, because you might be looking for reasons around you as to why your relationships keep failing when it could be as fundamental as you looking towards someone else for self-love. If a person feels he wasn't cared for or loved enough as a child, it would be a challenge for him to know how to love himself. It sounds like a paradox, for someone who doesn't know what love looks like to know how to love himself—so he looks for someone else to do it for him.

The rest of this book will also help you gain the skills needed to navigate relationships beyond what your parents showed you so you can put them into practice. In the meantime ...

Take control by understanding what gives you satisfaction and joy—either in solitude or in a romantic partnership. Assessing the rest of these self-growth pillars will help give you that understanding. Make a list of the things you enjoy doing solo and another of the things you enjoy doing with somebody special. If you're in a relationship but your sex life is in a rut, follow the advice scattered within all three rules discussed in this book. In addition, read authoritative, credible books about sexuality. Don't use YouTube, forums, and porn as your guide. Best of all, talk with your partner about each other's sexual desires and boundaries. Find the courage to talk about it. Sexual satisfaction is one of the perks of being in the Brave Hearts Brigade.

4.Financial state: At its very basic level, this pillar is about being able to live comfortably within your means. It's also about having savings and investments. And having enough for the luxuries that matter to you. How much money do you need for you to say you have a really good financial state? It all depends on you. Are you guided by others' judgments and expectations? Or do you go by what you personally value as worth having? For some, owning a mansion and frequent travel are true signs of financial success (even if they need to go deep into debt to get them). Others are content with a modest home, provided everyone there is happy—including the pets.

As Forrest Gump's mama said, "There's only so much fortune a man really needs, the rest is just for showing off." On the other hand, Gordon Gekko said, "Greed, for lack of a better word, is good. Greed is right. Greed works."

How do you assess the state of your financial pillar?
A) Really Good   B) Just Fine   C) Pretty Bad

If you answered A, kudos for being right where you are! If you chose B, I still have to say kudos! Not many people could declare themselves as having that level of satisfaction in money-matters. If you answered C, you're definitely not alone. Money is one of the top stressors in marriage and life in general. Couples tend to dodge discussing money matters for a variety of reasons—such as not wanting to impose or ruffle feathers, embarrassment over their debt, salary or spending habits. It could also be fear over how the other person might take it. The more they avoid talking about it, the more it causes friction and misunderstandings, resulting in a vicious cycle of fighting and dodging.

Take control by spending less and saving more. Even the tiniest changes will accrue to something bigger. Prioritize the elimination of debt. Budget better (using an app can help). Get to a place where you feel good about yourself, knowing you're doing your best to earn, spending wisely, and actively saving.

5.Occupational state: Closely related to the preceding pillar, this refers to pursuing careers or businesses in line with your personal goals and definition of success. How this differs from your financial state is that occupational satisfaction includes how you feel at the start and end of each workday, that is, whether you feel both challenged and inspired as each day progresses—this being distinct from the financial rewards. Many people stay in jobs they find miserable because it pays the bills. Others choose to follow their passion, content with little monetary gain but end up with a wealth of personal fulfillment and a sense of achievement.

Sometimes, the satisfaction doesn't come from only one occupation. For instance, I get a different kind of satisfaction from my advertising business than from my teaching and counseling careers, and yet another kind from my writing profession. It's important that you enjoy what you do, and that you do what you enjoy—and sometimes that enjoyment can come from a combination of endeavors.

When it comes to your occupational state, how do you feel?
A) Really Good   B) Just Fine   C) Pretty Bad

If you answered A, consider yourself blessed! For those who chose B or C, the common advice is to not settle. Keep working towards what you want. Improve your skills and increase your knowledge. Aim for optimal work-life balance and avoid over-working. Your relationships will benefit from it.

Take control by listing down your occupational goals and create a plan to reach them. It may not be necessary to change paths. It may simply be a matter of identifying what's holding you back or keeping you less than satisfied where you are and working on improving those conditions.

6.Environmental state: When you're at your favorite spot in your home, look around you. Do you like what you see? How it sounds? How it smells and feels? Your immediate surroundings affect your focus, your work, sleep, stress levels, and general wellness.

Go beyond that and consider your entire home and the neighborhood. That can have a huge influence on your overall life satisfaction, depending on what matters to you, such as if your environment reflects who you are, supports your sense of security and order, or how it contributes to your desire for tranquility or community.

The effects of your environmental state could be subconscious or personally tangible. How do you feel about it?

A) Really Good   B) Just Fine   C) Pretty Bad

If you answered A, then you're right where you ought to be! If you answered B and your priorities lie elsewhere, then embrace this feeling of contentment. If you chose C, you could take small steps to make some immediate improvements. Remember, the state of your environment can strongly affect your state of mind—and vice versa.

Take control by cleaning up your space. Bring more nature in. Improve the air quality around you. Spruce things up and decorate in ways that speak to your soul. For bigger changes, include this as a goal as you work on your financial state.

7.Intellectual state: This isn't about your educational attainment, mathematical prowess, or IQ score. Your intellectual growth encompasses all of your personal knowledge, whether you're book-smart, street-smart, well-versed in arts and culture, communication and social skills, have hobbies, or personal interests. Even now, as you read this book, you're expanding your self-knowledge and learning about relationships and romantic love.

It's important for any person, man or woman, to keep learning for the sake of learning, exploring new ideas, and engaging in activities and discussions that stimulate the mind. This makes you curious about your world, motivated to discover even more, and makes you a well-rounded and interesting person. More than that, keeping the mind engaged and challenged will help keep your mind robust well into your later years.

How do you feel about your intellectual growth lately?
A) Really Good   B) Just Fine   C) Pretty Bad

If you answered A, way to go! If you answered B or C, there are a lot of ways to broaden your intellectual horizon.

Take control by exploring new things that will broaden your mind. Read up on different topics—be it fiction of whatever genre, non-fiction, graphic novels, memoirs, or self-improvement books. You can take online courses and masterclasses on any topic that interests you. Visit museums, go to the theater. Watch documentaries. Have a pleasant exchange of ideas and discoveries within your social circle. Explore forms of entertainment that expose you to the unfamiliar.

8.Recreational state: If you're anything like me, you probably have a voice in your head that makes you uneasy about having an unoccupied moment. You get this nagging thought that you could be doing something more productive. There's always a deadline that needs to be chased. A meeting that shouldn't be delayed. A document that needs to be read, cleared, or commented on. Then during my down time, I start to think about what needs to be done around the house. And when that's finished and I have time for the gym, I tell myself I should at least be listening to an audiobook or podcast while doing those reps. Well, at least that's how it was for me for many decades.

I don't know what flicked the switch that shed light on my lack of leisure time. Yeah, I watched some shows or movies, attended events, and enjoyed some form of entertainment now and then, but these were mostly done because of other people in my life doing all the organizing, and I just went along with it. In other words, it was me attending to my social state and not my recreational state. What I lacked was time for my personal relaxation. I needed to do things for the purpose of purely easing the pressures of life on me!

It was only through my studies in psychology that I came to understand this often-overlooked slice in our wellness pie. It's the sweet slice of time not devoted to work, tasks, chores, or errands. It's time devoted to leisure and creativity—the missing piece that could help address many of our health issues, eliminate brain fatigue, lessen stress and boredom, give us better moods, and a lower heart rate.

But before you start crossing out all the mandated events and work commitments on your calendar, take note that there's a sweet spot when it comes to the quantity and quality of our leisure time. Several studies have shown that two to five hours of free time in a day is the Goldilocks region for positive effects on our well-being. Too little won't be enough to recharge us, leaving us emotionally drained. Too much free time, on the other hand, leads to decreased happiness because it undermines our sense of purpose.

Much like choosing between junk food and superfoods, what we spend our leisure time on is also vital. Simply immersing ourselves in a video game or the internet, or binge-watching Netflix doesn't quite do the job of revitalizing our spirit. The key to our joy is looking for experiences that offer us discovery, creativity, or make us feel rewarded. Seek out things that inspire awe, challenge, rejuvenate, change you in good ways, or give you stories to share.

Have you been engaging in enough creative endeavors, hobbies, or leisurely activities of the right kind?

How do you assess your recreational state?
A) Really Good   B) Just Fine   C) Pretty Bad

If you answered A, that's great! You probably wake up most mornings in a positive mood. If you answered B, it's only a matter of granting yourself more permission to seek leisurely escapes. If you chose C, it's time to redefine what 'having a good time' means for you—not as a wasted pursuit but as a necessary investment in your health.

Take control by unplugging and putting quality time for yourself on the calendar; time with no work to do, no obligations to fulfill. Yes, you need to plan it—"roughly." That is, set approximate goals such as a weekly tennis game or a monthly hike. Schedule them loosely so they stay on your to-do list without adding to the pressure of things you're obligated to fulfill. In other words, schedule with flexibility. Pick up a new (or neglected) hobby or sport. Create something. Learn to paint, play an instrument, or dance. Make yourself a tourist in nearby locales. Treat yourself by spending more time in nature. Keep in mind, the best thing to do with your free time is to use it—wisely.

9.Emotional state: This is about being comfortable with yourself as you recognize, regulate, and express your feelings to others. Young boys raised by caregivers who were empathetic and responsive to their needs are more comfortable dealing with their emotions growing up, unless society and culture forced them to camouflage or conceal them to avoid being shamed.

It's a tough one for most men who've been raised to deny their emotions—even to themselves. For these men, when a woman asks him the simple question, "What are you feeling?" it can render him clueless and speechless. Even though boys are born as emotional as girls, by the time they become men, most struggle to feel. A man can have intense physical sensations, say, an elevated heart rate, staggered breathing, sweaty palms—but ask him to name what he's feeling and verbalize it, he might have an easier time saying something in Klingon.

The ability to recognize your feelings, express them, and let yourself be vulnerable might be something alien to you now, or it might seem like a lost art. Other times, the trouble may be in processing or regulating them. You could have gotten so used to joking, intellectualizing, or arguing over issues, you've come to take that as "feeling" rather than masking them. Turning an emotional issue into a laugh, a brooding silence, or a heated discussion is not exactly opening one's heart to vulnerability.

Just like learning a language, emotional literacy is a skill than can be learned, practiced, and mastered—which is crucial to maintaining healthy relationships at home, at work, and in your social circle.

A widely accepted theory of emotions developed by psychologist Paul Ekman suggests we have six primary emotions that we all feel—regardless of gender, race, language, and culture. These are sadness, happiness, fear, anger, surprise, and disgust. A quick Google search of the term *emotion wheel* will expose you to a much wider range which will give you a hint of the emodiversity out there—the sheer variety and abundance of emotions that humans experience which most of us don't have the vocabulary with which to express them. Much less the skill to recognize and know what to do when confronted by most of them. Research has shown that being in possession of and in control of one's emodiversity can give rise to positive effects on mental and physical health, such as decreased depression and fewer doctors' visits.

In chapter 5, we'll be taking a deep dive into the topic of emotions when we tackle the third rule for men with the courage to love. In the meantime, what's your assessment of your current emotional state? Are you comfortable talking about your feelings?

How are you when it comes to dealing with strong emotions?

A) Really Good   B) Just Fine   C) Pretty Bad

If you answered A, then I'm sure you've got a good feeling about this! (Pun definitely intended.) If you went with B, that's still a good place to be, and with what you'll be learning in this section and in a later chapter about emotions, you'll be feeling even better about it in no time. If you answered C, you can take small steps immediately to get you to a better place.

Take control by overriding your kneejerk programming to dismiss, ignore, or suppress your feelings. Pay attention to them and be mindful of the physical sensations that come with each feeling. Allow yourself to acknowledge what you feel so you can identify it by name. (Do a quick image search for "emotion wheel" to increase your emotional vocabulary.) Resist shrugging aside the task of naming what you feel by just saying, "I don't know." The lady in your life will one day ask the question, "What are you feeling?" You need to be able to give an eloquent answer so you can start forging deeper emotional intimacy.

On a related note: Do your best to acquaint yourself with your triggers of negative feelings. Overreactions to otherwise neutral or innocuous statements are usually a telltale sign that an inner child got poked in the eye. For instance, if someone smiles and jokingly says, "It's your fault"—and though it was clearly said in good humor, you still feel either a spark of anger or annoyance or dread. *Triggers* are spotted when you notice that a response is disproportionate to the stimulus. When you perceive someone's shallow remark as a put-down, it could mean you're misinterpreting intentions. Take note and take charge of the moment and try to trace back in time to where that response came from. Maybe someone years ago had insulted you or accused you of something, and it resulted in a major emotional upheaval for you. Your subconscious mind might still be stuck in that moment that has been left unresolved. Knowing the source of your emotional responses helps you take better control in the present.

10.Spiritual state: Finally, we arrive at the pillar that will help you define your mission. This isn't about practicing a certain religion or belief system. It's about how you've personalized your life's journey and given it direction so as to obtain the most spiritual fulfillment. Your spiritual state is only as strong as how you've come to define your sense of purpose—the meaning of your life.

It's important for one's overall well-being to know that one is part of something bigger than himself. The Japanese call it *ikigai*. The French call it one's *raison d'etre*. For Costa Ricans, it's their *plan de vida*. By knowing your mission, you're able to make decisions and lead a life based on your core values. It shows your path to success while telling you what roads are best avoided.

Your mission is a very personal thing and varies widely from person to person. One's greatest spiritual fulfillment could be in making sure the Earth stays green and that nature gets all the respect it deserves. For another it could be to be God's example in being the best father to his children so he could influence others. Yet another could be spearheading advancements in the academe and helping devise new programs to improve education. It need not be huge or monumental. It could be as simple as spreading the joy of music or good food or basketball.

I was in third grade when I realized with extreme clarity that my mission was to be a writer. But what wasn't clear to me was what I would write about. It wasn't until I was already earning my bachelor's degree in journalism when I came to realize that I wanted to use my writing skills as a means to make this world a better place—but not as a journalist. After graduating, I eventually ended up with a career in advertising. Yet even as I earned my keep as a copywriter, I kept my eye fixed on another path where I would someday write about more meaningful things that would help improve the future of humankind. This book—written to help men have healthier and happier relationships—is just one drop in the bucket I aim to keep pouring my time and talent into until it's overflowing.

What about you? Have you come to identify your mission and are you living your life according to it? How do you feel about your spiritual state?

A) Really Good   B) Just Fine   C) Pretty Bad

If you answered A, I salute you! You're on the path that makes you part of something bigger. If you answered B, I hope you're on your way to further solidifying your vision and purpose. If you answered C, the good news is you've just finished this section of the book which was designed to help you take stock of the different pillars of your life, giving you a better perspective on things.

Take control by moving to the next two steps towards determining your mission: Taking stock of your strengths and taking charge of a change in the world.

STEP TWO: Take stock of your core values.

We've just finished going through all your self-growth pillars:

- Social – your relationships with family, friends, and communities

- Marital – how you feel about your present status

- Physical – how you care for your overall health, fitness, and appearance

- Financial – your present income streams, savings, and investments

- Occupational – how you feel about your career, vocation, or business

- Environmental – your immediate surroundings and the neighborhood

- Intellectual – the depth and breadth of your personal knowledge

- Recreational – how you use your free time wisely

- Emotional – your ability to identify, regulate, and express feelings

- Spiritual – what gives you a sense of greater purpose

Think about how you rated yourself in each one. Can you see a pattern that reveals the things that you prioritize or wish you were doing better at because they're important to you? These are directional signs towards your core values which were most likely the measures or standards by which you told yourself that you were doing really good, just fine, or pretty bad in any area of your life.

For instance, a man who's single with no serious relationship at the moment might say his marital state was really good if he valued independence, whereas someone who values marriage and family life would say this same situation was pretty bad.

When you take action on matters in a way that matches your core values, you'll tend to have a more positive outlook on life. Going back to the previous example, let's say you're a married man who values family life, and you got offered a career opportunity. It will give you a salary hike and have you traveling business class around the world most of the year. Everyone, including your wife, might encourage you to go for it, and so you accept. A few months in, you might wonder why you feel so stressed and dissatisfied despite the freedom, adventure, and financial gain that the new job has given you. Quite likely, it's because your spirit is hungry for time with your wife and children, and you wish you could be there to enjoy the backyard barbecues, weekend trips, and everyday bonding moments with them. You regret how FaceTime is just not the same as face-to-face time.

This goes to show how deeply important knowing your core values is. You could end up with every reason to be happy on the outside but be miserable on the inside. Finding joy, satisfaction, and contentment is only possible when the choices you make and the actions you take align with those values.

In addition, the overall quality of your romantic relationship strongly relies on the alignment of your core values with that of your partner. There are relationships that begin based on physical attraction, others are founded on how much each depends on the other. Values-based relationships have proven to be the most robust and are able to withstand the test of time. That's why being fully aware of your core values makes you far more able to find and then stay with a partner with whom you are truly compatible.

How to Identify Your Core Values

Consider the things you love, what you're passionate about, and what your strengths, skills, and interests are. Why do you suppose you gravitated there?

How do you spend your leisure time (or how would you have wanted to)? When you're at social events, what do you like talking about most? Do others see you as an authority on a particular subject? What are you most interested in and are curious to learn more about? What vision do you have that inspires you to do the things you're doing?

Once again, ask yourself why these became so. If you keep asking yourself why you decide, do, or prefer certain things, it will lead you down a path that shows you what you value most in life.

Asking "Why?" is crucial because that's how you get to the core. Let's say you're an avid book collector and your living room and den have overflowing bookshelves. Why? For Guy A, it could be because he values knowledge. To Guy B, it could be tradition because he grew up in a home that had walls covered with books. Guy C could be doing it to impress other people even though he hardly reads books at all.

When it comes to choosing schools for his children, Guy A will select the one best known for the quality of its education and graduates. Guy B will probably want his kids to go to the same school he did. Guy C might want the most impressive private school.

The *why* leads you to the core value behind the things you do or wished you'd done. What could these core values be? Here's a list of some common ones:

Adventure	Brotherhood	Creativity	Dignity
Excellence	Family	Generosity	Hard Work
Independence	Justice	Knowledge	Loyalty
Maturity	Novelty	Openness	Productivity
Quality	Responsibility	Success	Trust
Unity	Vitality	Wisdom	Youthfulness

This, by no means, is anywhere near a complete list of choices. Identifying your core values is a personal journey that requires introspection. Hopefully, because you've just finished your personal assessment of your self-growth pillars, you have a better understanding of your priorities and what's important to you. Now, you just need to know why.

Keep in mind that core values can change over time. For instance, a young man might value adventure and bravery. Then when he starts thinking of settling down, he may place more value on comfort and fidelity. And when he reaches the empty nest stage, he might put friendship and family above all. Through all these life stages, the importance he places on his health and financial security may be constant.

Generally, it would be good to focus on three to five core values at any given time in your life. Having too many could defeat the purpose of having these values guide you in making decisions with greater ease.Once you've uncovered your core values, hold on to these discoveries and take them to heart. Now, let's move on to the next and final step towards defining your mission.

STEP THREE: Take charge of a change in the world.

"So you've had a good look inside?" Ethan Hunt asks as we exit the house and take a deep breath of the outside air. He reminds us of what he'd said when we first met up with him, that every man needs to ask himself: *What is my mission in life?* What matters most to him? What does he want to devote his life to the most? In knowing this, the woman he chooses to spend the rest of his life with should appreciate and support it, so that the two of them together become Mission: Compatible.

Ethan turns to us with a serious glint in his eyes. "Determining your mission begins with a simple thought: What does the world need?"

"A helluva lotta stuff," you answer.

Ethan grins and nods. "But you can narrow it down by looking at it from the perspective of what the world needs that *you* can do something about." Once again, he thrusts a finger at your chest.

Your mission lies at the intersection of:

• Your strengths and aptitudes

• Your core values

• The needs of the world

(If you can get paid for it too, that's a bonus.)

As mentioned earlier, this mission need not be spectacular or daunting. Of course, there's nothing stopping you from aiming to end world hunger, advance space exploration, or help humankind achieve immortality. Your life's purpose needs to matter to you; it's not about impressing others. What matters is that you go for it.

One's mission could spring from a very personal interest that, at first glance, might seem trivial but in the end, can prove life-changing for those touched by it. Let's say, for instance, that in your self-growth exercise, you realized that you spend most of your leisure time playing tennis and that this is a talent and a skill you have and something you're also passionate about.

After a bit of soul searching, you now also know that a couple of your core values turn out to be fitness and camaraderie, so you got to understand why you ended up enjoying tennis so much.

From this context, you can look at what the world needs, and you conclude that more people should discover a love for tennis because it's been proven to improve our social life and is one of the top sports that help people live longer.

You can then make that your mission! To help people live happier, healthier, longer lives by spreading the love for tennis. You can keep your day job but be more motivated with this new purpose that you can pursue on the side. At this point, you can start making other decisions and changes in your life that will align with this mission. That includes the decisions you make when it comes to the kind of woman you want to spend the rest of your life with. If you intend to live a life devoted to the love of tennis, then it seems not the ideal thing to date women with no appreciation for sports.

If your mission is to become an exemplary father and a role model of parenting, then you might want to make sure you find a wife who will share that grand vision of family life. If your purpose is to spread the word on the best tourist sites of the world, then it would be a bad idea to become attached to a homebody. If your goal is to make sure no animal is ever hurt or abandoned, then it would be tricky to become involved with someone who has a phobia of dogs.

So go ahead, look inside yourself. Find your purpose—because every single one of us needs to be part of something bigger than ourselves. And life would be so much easier if we found ourselves in a relationship with someone who supports that mission—and whose life's mission we can support just as whole-heartedly in return.

A House Made for Self-Love

At the beginning of this section, I'd asked you to think of yourself as a house with many rooms. We've had a grand tour of that house, assessed the state of each room, and allowed it to guide you in identifying your core values and your mission.

Now think of that house as a grand mansion that was gifted to you, left under your care, for you to keep enjoying. The entire house is you. It's priceless. Yet sometimes, you could end up fixated on a room or two that need refurbishment and forget to celebrate those areas that make you proud. Oftentimes, the reasons for our dissatisfaction may not even be the state we are *factually* in but are more because of "echoes in the hallway"—voices in our head that tend to see things from a dark and negative perspective despite the sunshine streaming in from the rest of our lives.

This entire section has been about self-awareness that will lead to complete self-acceptance—of every single room in the house that is you. It's a house that you control. And by inspiring you to take control of what you can, I hope it's clear that self-acceptance doesn't mean accepting that the worst-you-are-now is the best you can be. Self-acceptance means seeing yourself in bright light, with pure honesty, and realizing—perhaps for the first time—that this is your situation now, and you accept it without blame. And now, you can take better care of it—with self-love.

What is self-love?

I realize the term self-love can cause some men to recoil, cringe, or roll their eyes. If you're one of them, then I ask you to use your newfound emotional mindfulness to understand why you might feel that way. Is there something in your past that may have led you to think that loving oneself is not dignified or isn't something a man needs? If others failed to show you the tenderness you needed to feel loved, then begin by giving yourself the kindness, forgiveness, and appreciation you've always deserved.

2023 research by the University of Pittsburgh's Amanda Forest and her colleagues suggests that what makes or breaks a good relationship can be an individual's self-esteem, affecting how easily partners share their feelings and react to each other's needs. That's how important loving yourself is. A Brave Heart is someone who has taken stock of all aspects that make up who he is, is taking charge of what makes up his identity, and has gained the courage to share his whole being with his partner.

It's important that self-love is not mistaken for egoism or egocentricity. This isn't about being entitled or expecting others to simply admire, obey, or serve you. Nor is self-love about defining oneself as "enough"—to mean that he has no need for others to navigate through life.

Self-love is about being confident that you can enter somebody's space and be accepted for who you are and stand up to protect your boundaries if others cross them. Being *enough* means you are fully aware of all the bits and pieces that make up the total you—and that you're in control of all those aspects that make you *whole*.

You are enough—and spending time alone with just yourself, for yourself, feels good.

There's a lot of advice out there on how to show yourself this love—such as treating yourself or buying gifts for yourself. Journaling is another way you can express gratitude for your days, set down goals, and give yourself a pat on the back when you achieve them. But these can all end up superficial without the reality of that inner love. It will be like giving someone a sip of water when what they need is a constant supply of clean water, day after day.

The reason I took you through the exercise of those ten self-growth pillars—the many rooms of the house that represented you—was for you to love *you* first—and understand *why*.

Accepting yourself is knowing yourself—your greatest weaknesses and your greatest strengths—and playing the cards you've been dealt the best way you can so you have every chance of winning. Nobody's perfect. It's such a cliché and yet many people fail to accept their own imperfections.

Finding joy lies in how you deal with the past, present, and future. Let go of your past regrets, resist comparing yourself to others in the present, and focus your efforts on doing your best moving forward. Treat yourself with kindness. Be forgiving of yourself as you strive to do better wherever you can.

Practice gratitude for every single thing that's great about you. It's often the case that we get so fixated on the one thing we don't have and fail to celebrate every other wonderful thing in our lives. Accept the entirety of you with love and respect. Then when you look in the mirror, give two thumbs up and tell that guy you see, "You're doing great."

A Short Pause in Our Hero's Journey

At this point, Ethan asks us to move over to the side of the road and take a breather under the shade of a tree. He has us open up our Knapsack of Knowledge and review what we've picked up along the way.

As if given your own *Mission: Impossible*, you were tasked to find your own mission in life on your way to finding *Mission: Compatible*. He hopes you've come to realize that the first step towards recognizing someone compatible is understanding yourself.

After assessing yourself through the ten self-growth pillars, identifying your top three to five core values, and finding a mission that you can be part of in changing the world, you are now far more self-aware than when you started on this journey.

Take a deep breath and sense how good that feels—to know that what defines you as a man is not something external or what other people expect of you. What defines you as a man is how you define yourself.

You are enough. Meaning, you don't need a *Mission: Compatible* woman to complete who you are in your eyes and in other people's judgment. Though, as a reader of this book, it can be assumed that your heart still desires a woman who complements your world.

"Why?" you may wonder. That's where we're headed next on this journey of discovery. When you're ready, buckle up that knapsack and let's move on towards a deeper understanding of why—despite being complete—a man still feels the need for a special woman in his life.

Why Do You Love Her?

One of the first psychologists to tackle the concept of self-love is Eric Fromm who wrote, "Love of others and love of ourselves are not alternatives. On the contrary, an attitude of love toward themselves will be found in all those who are capable of loving others." Self-love, therefore, is necessary before anyone can love another.

In other words, the primary rule is to consciously and actively love yourself. Because whatever relationship you choose to go for will be determined by *what you believe you deserve*. Elevate your self-perception and you elevate the choices that you make and that will encompass your friendships, activities, aspirations—including what you believe you deserve in your romantic relationship and what you are able to give. Let's recap that last part: *Elevate what you believe you deserve in your romantic relationship and what you are able to give*. Value yourself highly then you won't settle for less. Be the man who believes he deserves a high-value woman.

Which brings us to a question few men bother to ponder. Why does a man seek to be in a relationship with a woman? After all, he was raised to be the King of Independence. The one who brought home the bacon and looked after the safety of others. And with everyone knowing what the oldest profession is—plus the way things are going with modern-day dating—nearly all cultures have been highly forgiving of men who get sex with no strings attached, no commitments, or no promises required.

So why does a man need a woman and a committed relationship in his life? The reflex response many young men have is to get quick and easy access to sex. If that's your answer, then you probably haven't come across the research published in 2019[11] which revealed that married individuals tended to score lower than others on sexual communication, sexual self-esteem, and sex frequency. Data shared by Statista reveals that as of 2022, 33.1% of married baby boomers in the United States live in a sexless marriage, so do 22.9% from Generation X, and 7.4% of millennials. These numbers tell us that a romantic commitment is no guarantee of that regular dose of sex you're looking for. You might end up getting more by staying single with a bunch of dating apps. (Not that I'm prescribing it.)

The sciences will tell you that humans are biologically polygamous and culturally monogamous. That is, we are not designed by nature to mate for life; the hormonal mix that stirs up the crazy-in-love feelings last only six months to three years. After that, it's a decision you make to stay. It's a combination of civilization, religion, societal norms, and the strong influence of emotions that have elevated monogamy to an essential ingredient for a stable, long-term relationship.

If you examine that through the prism of body, heart, and mind, it looks like this: the body is polygamous, the heart desires monogamy, and the mind is what makes the choice between the two.

So what drives that choice to stay committed to one woman?

Up until a few decades ago, raising a family together could have been a major reason. According to the U.S. Census Bureau, more than 40% of households back in 1970 were headed by married parents with children under the age of 18. By 2021, that number had fallen to 17.8%. Another survey conducted in 2018 found that less than one in three adults in the U.S. believe that being married is essential to live a fulfilling life, and only 36% believe that having kids is essential to fulfillment. What was viewed as most essential? 65% said it was having a rewarding job—that's more than twice as many people who said that marriage was essential.

Within a few decades, a lot has changed. Entering a committed relationship to raise a family is no longer seen as essential to a fulfilling life as it used to be.

So, is it not about fulfillment, in a personal sense, but more about "having it all" in the eyes of others? I offer this as a possibility because of the surprising reason some people give for choosing a partner or for staying with one. *We look great on Instagram.* Or variations thereof. When others tell them they look great together. Or that they seem like a perfect couple. Or that he hit the jackpot and might not get another woman that pretty.

Men have clung to unhappy relationships for fear of disappointing others who approve of his partner and their relationship. It's as though staying committed to this woman simply added to his credentials, because a beautiful woman by his side completed his image of being the guy who had it all—an admirable career, lots of money, time to travel, nice cars, and a house with a beautiful wife and kids waiting inside. But you probably know of at least one man who has achieved every item on that list but confesses to still feeling empty and unhappy. So having a long-term relationship with a woman just for display could either lead to a dissolution of that union or him growing old lonely, despite "having it all."

A more common answer I hear about why a man seeks a romantic relationship is to fulfill his need to be needed. But that's a fundamental need everyone has, regardless of gender. And yet there are many who choose to stay single and are happy. Becoming a monk or joining the clergy can fulfill one's need to feel that need. Being a single parent or an aunt or uncle who cares for their nephews and nieces can get that feeling too. Even people who volunteer to save homeless animals and the Earth from pollution can feel especially needed. And as proven by the survey cited above, having a fulfilling career works rather well too. A man doesn't have to be in a romantic relationship to feel needed.

So let me fine-tune my question to something more specific: Why do you seek to be in a long-term, committed, romantic relationship beyond getting sex, kids, credentials, and a need to feel needed?

Let's pause for a moment here. Put down this book and give it some thought. *Why do you?*

Through the years, I've witnessed the evolution of the answer to that question. I've been teaching university students for the past two decades and have had the opportunity to ask that question of young men in my advertising classes. These are men in their late teens and early twenties, generally unjaded, possibly still idealistic, and having mostly their home life as a basis for their answers.

I challenged them to write a marketing brief for a planet inhabited only by heterosexual men. They had to sell the idea of "importing" women for the prospect of marriage wherein sex and raising kids was not in the picture. (Do note that I had the women do the same exercise in reverse; that is, market men to an all-female planet. In both worlds that I made up for the exercise, storks delivered the babies to their doorstep.) The all-male groups needed to come up with a woman's unique selling proposition (USP) which the target market couldn't get from their current relationships with other heterosexual men.

Granted, these conditions require an extreme suspension of disbelief, but it was an exercise designed to teach advertising students the power of a consumer desire when it matches a product promise. And therein lay the challenge. Because, if a planet has prospered, populated by heterosexual men alone fulfilling all the essential roles of society, it implied it didn't need to import another gender. As an ad agency, their job was to make men want something they believed they didn't need. Just like how Apple convinces people who are doing fine with a desktop computer, a laptop, and a smartphone that they need an iPad too.

Now, how does this fictitious setup become relevant to the readers of this book who aren't interested in honing their advertising skills? Let's transpose the scenario into a closer-to-home counterpart—so instead of going to a galaxy far, far away, let's go back in time to a period not so, so long ago.

Imagine traveling back to a time when all men believed their greatest roles were to provide for those who depended on them and to protect the weak. This meant that the women they chose to "import" into their lives would rely on them for all their basic and major necessities in life (because she was usually incapable of getting hired for a job or of getting far in a man's world). This also meant that the women would be dependent on the men for their place of residence, safety, and security. The men spent their days at work, oblivious to whatever transpired at home because there was no internet or mobile phones or instant messaging apps. It was extremely rare for a landline phone call to be made for household concerns unless it was a dire emergency. At the end of the day, the man might choose to pass by a pub after work, and when he arrived home, the food was ready, the place was spic and span, and the children smelling fresh despite spending the day in school or playing out in the yard. The wife might be in a dour mood, but it didn't concern him much, because if he wanted to "do the act" later that night, she would oblige. If, on the other hand, he no longer found sex pleasurable with her but still valued her as the caring homemaker and mother of his kids, then he could find other ways to satisfy himself. There were other women out there willing to play that role despite them knowing he was already married. And society was largely forgiving of men who strayed.

Now, imagine that a glitch in time suddenly transported all these men into their future—which is our today. They look around them and see women working side-by-side with men from entry level positions to the very top in nearly all corners of the working world. Today's woman is often neither dependent on nor subservient to men and no longer lives in constant fear that she will be harmed by one of them. This has given her the courage to speak up and debate with him, correct him, and even treat him rudely in front of others—as well as in private. When in a relationship, women can easily say "no" and demand for more time and attention from her partner, including help with the housework and childcare—or else she would throw a fit. And unlike before, when hitting a woman or having a string of extra-marital affairs was more or less tolerated, society (including strangers) could now shame a man for these and lesser offenses instantly, publicly, globally, with just a few taps of their thumbs on a screen.

When the men from the past were asked by future-folk, "Would you still wish to marry a woman of this day?" They look perplexed and asked right back, "Why would men want to? What on Earth is in it for them?"

Answering that question, from another perspective, was the very task I had asked my male advertising students to explore.

In the early 2000s, the male students' answer for a woman's USP, as to why men should 'import' her into their all-male planet, often started out along the lines of having someone around who was better at doing the housework—which I told them they could get by hiring a houseboy and a cook. There were also suggestions of a USP that women would help them be better at taking care of themselves—something, I said, even a male nanny or "manny" can do. As the years went by, the USP shifted to having someone nice to come home to—which I said they could get with a Labrador Retriever. They would then refine the answer to companionship, having someone to come home to at the end of the day whom they can relax and talk with—which I said Chandler and Joey also got as F.R.I.E.N.D.S.

Up until a few years ago, it still took quite a bit of soul-searching for these young men in my advertising class to find a proposition truly *unique* to having a serious relationship with a woman. Recently though,

Gen Z men have found it much easier to come up with that rare promise (perhaps indicating a shift in how younger men perceive the role their mothers have in their fathers' lives). Yet no matter how long it took, invariably, year after year, the students landed on variations of the same answer: Softness. Tenderness. A safe place to be vulnerable.

What this told me was that these men were tired of always being jabbed—physically, mentally, and emotionally. Each one wanted a reprieve from always being on his toes, prepared to defend or steel himself against ridicule, mockery, or shame from other men. Even camaraderie came with a shortage of tenderness, warm compliments, and a soothing embrace.

Men need women because it's a hard world out there where they constantly need to prove their manhood, their worth, and their status to other men. In the privacy of his heart, a man clings to a hope that there remains one bastion of peace where he can be unconditionally loved and desired—just for being himself. It's a fortress that guards the one place where his heart and pride are safe. It's a place where the woman he loves waits.

For her to not know this can be a great source of sadness for a man; especially if she becomes a constant source of blame, shame, and challenges to his sense of self-worth.

We've now arrived at the point where I get to ask you for your answers.

- Why do you seek to be in a long-term, committed, romantic relationship beyond getting sex, kids, credentials, and a need to feel needed?

- Given your answer to that question, is the woman you have in your heart, mind, and life now the right one for you?

If you gave a quick and unabashed "Hell, yeah!" in response to the second question, I'm profoundly happy for you. If, on the other hand, you replied with a hearty "Hell no!" then I hope you understand better what it is you are worth and what you deserve. There are times we find ourselves holding on to something that no longer serves us, and it's particularly difficult to leave even an unhappy relationship because of psychological barriers and fears—like "What will others think?" or "What if I end up alone?" Being stuck in an unhappy relationship that lacks a sense of friendship and partnership, shared values, and mutual respect can be detrimental to our health. The anxiety, chronic stress, and depression this elicits can have profound effects on our mental, emotional, and even physical well-being. Good health and a long, fulfilling life go hand-in-hand with happiness.

One of the top reasons why people stay on in unhappy relationships is the fear of being alone. And also, the fear of the pain and conflict involved in the process of breaking up. One must realize that settling for a difficult relationship keeps you from finding a healthier one that will give you the love, happiness, and well-being you deserve. It helps knowing that what you learn from this relationship can help you find fulfillment in the next one—if you believe that being in a relationship is something you really need and want right now. It's true that it means entering the dating scene again, which is daunting at any age. But part of being a Brave Heart is finding the courage to step out there and to be open to finding the relationship that's right for you.

If you answered, "I'm not sure," or "Maybe?"—the next section will help clarify matters for you. Seeing things in a new light could help bridge the gap that's keeping you from answering "Yes." Continue reading and get more insights into the feminine mind and pointers on how to improve your relationship.

Now that we've gotten the answers we came here to find, Ethan Hunt nods with approval, stating his mission: complete. He bids us farewell and points us down the road to the next leg of our journey—where we'll get to try our hand at some good old-fashioned detective work.

Be Sherlock Holmes. Ask the Right Questions and Find the Right Woman.

Rule No. 1: Know Who You Love—and Why

We gather inside a quaintly furnished country cabin along our journey. Sherlock Holmes greets us with a solid observation. "It's elementary, my dear man. Getting married or moving in together won't magically transform sad singles into a joyful pair."

Asked to further explain Rule No. 1, Holmes says, "Knowing who you love—and why. That rule has many sides to it. You knowing you, and you knowing her—*and* why you love her."

Holmes puts on his signature deerstalker hat. "Let's all put on our thinking caps, shall we? Take your pick." He gestures towards a wooden rack filled with hats of different sorts: newsboy caps, flat caps, berets, and beanies.

He strikes a match to light his pipe as you select your hat. "How much do you know about the woman you love?" You dig inside your head for information besides what most other people can glean from your partner's social media. Holmes puffs on his pipe and stares at you as you put on the hat you've chosen. "Have you asked her the questions you've asked yourself? Those which helped you understand yourself better?"

You cough as the cloud of smoke in front of his face dissipates.

"What did love look like to her in her childhood?" Holmes asks. "What was her relationship like with her parents? How did her mother show love to her father? How did her father show love to her mom?"

He walks towards a table, lays down his pipe, and picks up a Rubik's cube. "Much like a woman, wouldn't you say?" he asks, brandishing the puzzle. "Many sides. Many permutations. Takes a bit of figuring out."

A Woman's Many Permutations

Everyone may find a certain woman clever, charming, and bubbly to have as company. But after you become a couple, it may seem like she's transformed. You wonder what it was you did that caused the change. That's one explanation worth exploring. Though it's also possible that it's something related to her past.

Smart, beautiful, and fun-loving women can end up acting cold and distant in a relationship because their parents, even if they'd remained married, hadn't displayed warmth or tenderness to one another while in front of their children. These women could end up feeling uncomfortable receiving that kind of devotion from you—because to them, it seems unnatural and unfamiliar. They might even find your caring ways "unmanly" because it's not something they ever saw from their fathers. Not ever having seen it before in real life, it could make reciprocating feel artificial to them because they're just making it up as they go along.

Another possibility could be that of a smart, beautiful, and fun-loving woman who ends up needy, clingy, and dependent in a relationship because of a different core wound from childhood. Maybe her parents had divorced early, and this could have left her with a subconscious fear of abandonment having had her comfortable "bubble of foreverness" burst at an early age. Or maybe she used to be close to a parent who suddenly withdrew their attention when that parent got too busy at work or had to travel constantly. Or maybe she had parents who scolded her a lot or only took notice of her when she had stellar achievements in school but otherwise didn't show any interest in her everyday life.

There are many possible reasons why a woman behaves differently with you than how she is in front of others. And many of these reasons may have little to do with you and more to do with hidden emotional wounds from childhood or past romantic relationships. Asking questions gets you to see these wounds that are still bleeding or seemingly healed but are still hurting.

Get to know her well so you can empathize better. Knowing about your woman's emotional scars helps you navigate her heart, so you become sensitive to her pain and help her heal. Rather than being at the mercy of her moods and whims, you get to anticipate the twists and turns of the relationship. You get to lead the tango.

Ideally, she would do the same for you. She, too, can help you heal when you show her your vulnerability. But that depends on her emotional maturity—which you can uncover, gauge, and nurture the more you ask questions, listen, and get to understand each other better.

One of the things you need to decipher is why she treats you the way she does. What role do you think she takes on when it comes to loving you?

Her Motherly Role

Sherlock Holmes had good reason to use a Rubik's cube for his metaphor. It will serve us well as we talk about a woman's many sides.

The role women are most familiar with is that of a mother—even when she doesn't have kids. It's the role she portrayed while playing with her dolls. And if her primary caregiver had been her mother, it's the version of womanhood she had been most exposed to growing up, thus making it the easiest to model.

Mom is the mentor who showed her it's good to notice everything there is to notice, correct everything less than perfect, and remember everything that others forget. Unfortunately, without a woman realizing it, this kind of "corrective attention" could end up being her language of expression when showing love to her partner—because that was how her mother expressed her love to her family. It's driven by a notion that it's part of her duty to ensure everyone is being the best they can be, sometimes to the point of making her man feel like he is the child who needs to be disciplined.

Because this is the most dominant persona that a woman may subconsciously end up modeling, I'll need to dwell on this for a bit. The ease by which a woman could slip into the role of mother to her man is almost second nature because even men tend to start relating to her like he was her son without him realizing it.

A Man and His Mother's Role

Think back to how you were raised by your mother (or primary female caregiver.) This was your first experience on how to relate with women, and it's what will end up comfortable and "normal" for you—whether that relationship felt great, just tolerable, or far from ideal. Because you grew up used to that kind of interaction, it left you with a sense of familiarity, even if it was distant, chaotic, cold, confusing, or even toxic—it's what you became accustomed to.

If your mother generally neglected your emotional or physical needs, you might have grown up very independent and not wanting to rely on anyone, so you keep your partner emotionally distant. If you were doted on or spoiled by your mother, there's a huge chance you ended up expecting the same kind of special treatment from your wife. If, on the other hand, you used to be the one constantly helping your mother out, then you might always be ready to take care of all your woman's needs, from handling a lot of the housework to helping her with other needs that your mother used to rely on you for, like driving, doing groceries, or carrying things around. If your mother wasn't much of a decision maker and you used to have to step in to advise her—or go against her will—then you might see yourself as the one responsible for making most of the decisions in the house and taking charge of getting things done. A very controlling mother might also have left you feeling resigned to have a nagger for a wife—or fearful of ending up with one.

If you could relate to any of these, you were conditioned to consider that as the norm, so quite likely your first few relationships will be modeled after this, until you make a conscious effort to break free from that pattern. This is attributed by John Gottman, psychologist and researcher, to a phenomenon known as imprinting, wherein a child becomes conditioned at a very early age to be attracted to a certain parental personality type and the kind of love and care that was or wasn't given.

In other words, outside of the bedroom, it's highly likely that the relationship you have with your partner most closely resembles the relationship you had with your mother or primary caregiver. You gravitated there or are staying there because of familiarity, not necessarily because it's a source of joy. Related to this is the topic of attachment styles which are shaped in our early youth; we will be touching on that a few sections down the road to give you a better idea of how they affect your relationships. For now, let's focus on how a woman's motherly role could be affecting how she relates with you. And vice versa.

Much the same as you having entered this relationship with patterns from your past, so did your partner. If she grew up with a healthy, nurturing relationship with her mother, then she should have the empathy and emotional robustness to be able to respond to your emotional needs in a supportive manner. In contrast, if she grew up emotionally famished, then she could end up feeling more comfortable in a relationship that keeps you in that famished state, because that's what's familiar to her. Similarly, if you were the one who grew up with your emotional needs unmet, you might find yourself drawn to women who are clingy because they hold the unspoken promise of giving you the attention you never got as a child. So, once in a while, a bit of baby talk or a mischievous little-boy act might slip out, seeking some nurturing, understanding, or tender caring from the new woman in your life—the kind of attention the juvenile you didn't get enough of and is now seeking from someone willing to give it.

Allow me to digress a moment and expound on that topic. Let's set aside the Rubik's cube for a couple of minutes and have a quick "juvenile" discussion.

Let's Talk About Baby Talk

Find a romantic couple talking in the high-pitched voice grownups use with infants. Add the use of pet names like wuvvy-dovey and woogie-pooh. Then toss in the singsong tone of a toddler you can't help but cuddle. What have you got? Baby talk. For some, the sound of it makes their toes curl. For others, it's a sign of a couple in wuv ... I mean, love.

Baby talk, per se, between romantic partners is not a cause for concern. A study from the Kinsey Institute states that two-thirds of couples use baby talk with each other. It might have evolutionary origins because research shows that the practice cuts across cultures. Psychologists say that it's healthy and can be indicative of a secure relationship because it signifies a willingness to show vulnerability.[12] It's also proven that using pet names like "bunny," "sweetie pie," or "honey bun," predicted greater relationship satisfaction for both husbands and wives because it's an endearing yet quick way to elicit the affection you need.

There is one anecdotal study,[13] however, that shows a difference in responses between hearing a partner declare one's love followed by a pet name (I love you, honey) versus their name (I love you, Chris) or nothing at all (I love you). Saying, "I love you, honey," triggered a quicker reciprocation, but saying, "I love you, Chris," brought on a slower subtle sensation with an undercurrent of desire.

If your significant other is one to use pet names, I personally advice the use of those which still comfortably sound like an adult, like McDreamy, Handsome, or Love—to keep the mental picture she has of her man a "man," as opposed to a stuffed toy she might have had in preschool, like Shmoopy, Boo-boo, or Pookie Head. To look at it from another perspective: When do you find a man or woman most desirable and sexy? It's when they act like an adult. Labeling them with something that says the opposite sends the wrong signal. Unfortunately, I don't have large-scale research and am only going by anecdotal feedback to support this suggestion, but there are men who feel embarrassed or uncomfortable when given these childish pet names. So if you like it, then let her know. If you don't, it's a good idea to tell her.

I must admit though that I instinctively flinch when I hear a woman call her partner "Babe" because of the subliminal signal I imagine that it sends her brain—and his—on how she's supposed to treat him. For the same reason, I wouldn't consider it a wise thing to start calling each other "Mommy" or "Daddy." One client of mine who was assessing why he'd lost feelings of sexual attraction towards his wife told me, "I look at her and all I see is the mother of my children." Similarly, I'd discourage a man acting like a needy, hard-headed, or servile little boy with his partner—even in jest or as a playful way of seeking affection—because it provokes her to treat him like her son.

Being emotionally vulnerable, meaning being honest about your feelings, is different from acting like a child. You can weep in a moment of frailty and still be very much an adult coping with life. Putting on a kiddie-cute act to get her attention is something else; it puts her in Mother Mode. If you want to keep seeing each other as sexual partners, I suggest that you be conscious about it and nip this habit in the bud, because it's going to be difficult to unlearn this mother-and-son dynamic after it sets in. Talk with each other and find out how this way of interacting affects you both.

Is She a Spender or a Saver?

I knew years before I got married that the number one thing married couples fight about is money. And so, long before I even met the person I would exchange "I dos" with, I already vowed something I wouldn't do: Fight about money.

As I will say repeatedly in this book, avoiding topics that are needed to be discussed is one big mistake; and it's a mistake I obviously made. That's the essence of being part of the Brave Hearts Brigade today. It's finding the courage to have those difficult conversations, no matter the minefield that you know could be waiting for you up ahead. Because there's a right way of moving forward so nothing explodes in your face.

As part of Rule No. 1, which is knowing who you love, when it comes to the matter of money management, you'll need to find out if you and your partner are similar or opposites in your financial personalities. Is she a spender or a saver? What about you? You'll need to figure out how the two of you will do the tango gracefully through life if you're dancing in opposite directions around your funds.

Research provides evidence supporting a few things couples need to set in place to keep the money music playing harmoniously. Wherever you're at in your relationship, it's never too late to add some new steps to a couple's financial choreography.

- **Schedule financial coffee breaks.** Or money talk time. Or budget burger dates. Whatever you call it, make it a regular tête-à-tête about money matters. It could be monthly or quarterly. But don't do what I did. We sat down once to divvy up expenses when we were newlyweds—and never again. After that, it became half-expressed resentments and disappointments over expenses through the years (because I'd mistakenly thought not fighting was the safer thing to do). Do the smart thing and make it a regular date so it's planned for and remains consistent. Setting it at the start of every month enables you to adjust your budgets based on the particular needs up ahead.

- **Get to know each other's financial personalities.** Do you prefer to spend on grand vacations and luxury items, but she would rather put more money into savings and investments? Are you aware of each other's debt profile? How many credit cards do each of you have? It's important that you both come clean about any bad spending habits or any personal or family issues that could eat into your budgets. Being open and honest will help you accomplish the next step better.

- **Agree on goals and plans.** Your long-term financial goals as a couple should also be something discussed and revisited. These revolve around your priorities such as the house you live in, raising children, how much you want to travel, and what your dreams for retirement are. If one or both of you still have debts to deal with, you'll need to examine debt payoff strategies and agree on how you want to handle things moving forward. Caring for extended family can also become a sore spot. What happens when one of you constantly needs to give financial assistance to parents or siblings? There's also such a thing as "financial infidelity," when one partner has money squirreled away in a secret bank account or spends on luxury items without letting the other know. Sometimes, simply agreeing to be transparent and asking for permission could be enough to solve any issues. Other times, it could mean setting a cap. Discuss what works for both of you.

- **If you haven't yet, open a joint account**. Numerous research studies have proven that couples who pool their finances improve the quality of their relationship over time,[14] and how those who do the opposite (i.e. keep their money in separate accounts or hybrids of partly joint-partly separate) exhibit a decline.[15] The reasons cited include how pooling your earnings invites open and constant communication which keeps the couple's financial goals aligned. This helps build a sense of being part of a team which in turn improves how the couple feels about how they handle money together.

Be wary of any power play that might happen when one partner has significantly more money than the other. It could happen that the one who brings in more wants to make all the decisions, causing a buildup of resentment in their partner. Conversely, the one contributing less might go about life assuming their partner is perfectly all right with the arrangement and not realize that there's a mound of discomfort—or bitterness—silently growing around the situation.

It's important to keep in mind that you're part of a team, and as the conditions of your life together change, so should the dynamics of your financial teamwork. Sometimes, one team member's contributions might be going unseen and unappreciated because they come in the form of heartwarming deeds instead of cold cash. (In a later section, we'll talk about the "invisible load." It's the household planning, thinking, and organizing that often goes unnoticed. If one were to monetize that mental and emotional load, you'd realize that not all work that helps keep the home afloat involves physical labor and comes with a salary).

All that being said, it needs to be noted that there are many factors in play that could make what works for the majority not ideal for others. The advice I've culled shouldn't be considered a cure-all for every situation; there needs to be a certain level of emotional stability and mutual trust in place.

So what role does your partner play in your team's money management? Are you okay with that, and is she all right with yours?

Women's Other Roles

I'm picking up Sherlock Holmes' metaphorical cube again as I continue my discussion of women's many colorful sides and turn it so we can have a look at another dominant female presence in women's lives: teachers.

As of 2022, women made up 75% of all teachers in America. In Europe, this extends to over 90% for pre-primary and primary years of school. The highest share of female teachers in the pre-primary school level is in East and Southeast Asia at 97%. Once again, she has a wealth of female role models who show her that it's part of caring to correct, guide, and ... well, teach. Which could lead a woman to use that behavior as a means of showing her nurturing side—that of trying to help make you a better man by pointing out a faster, smarter, safer, cheaper, way of doing just about anything. It might feel disrespectful of your own judgment or a display of her lack of trust in you. But because she didn't feel offended when her teachers did these to her, she may not be sensitive to how it makes you—a grown man—feel. She may even wonder why you would take offense or why your ego gets in the way when all she's trying to do is contribute to making life better, faster, safer, easier, or whatever.

With several twists of the Rubik's cube, we glimpse other dimensions of a woman.

There's also her stereotypical role of multi-tasker. Remember Kro-ah, the mother of Brongk from the caveman era? Women today still have the same inclinations—that of heeding a sense of dread that if she forgets or overlooks something, the village will go up in smoke. If you're not convinced that this is still how women think, then just consider the recent Oscar-award winning movie, *Everything Everywhere All at Once*. The title alone, reflective of what the lead female character thinks about, says it all.

If she's a working woman, then there's a huge chance you're also familiar with the boss or leader hat she wears, which she often forgets to hang by the door when she gets home. After which, she dons the additional hat of homemaker—thus turning her into the homemaker-boss, which, in case you still haven't realized, is a role the modern woman would rather share and not have men assume is hers to claim.

That's quite a lot of roles and hats all coming together in one person, and this might have been keeping you on your toes, wondering who you'll be coming home to at the end of every day. But don't worry. This is where the tips for communicating better, discussed under Rule No. 3, should come in. That chapter down the road will give ideas on how to relate better with her mothering, multi-tasking, teacher, and boss-lady tendencies without you needing to retreat into your cave, never to come out again.

A woman has many other roles, of course. That of daughter, sister, aunt, confidante, tutor, friend, etc., and it's quite possible that you never considered what roles you've been hoping she'd play in your life—and if she'd be okay with them. The role of mother to your children (how soon and how many); the housemate who shares the house chores and the bills; secretary, if you count on her keeping track of schedules, appointments, and meaningful dates for the both of you; therapist, if you want her to listen to your issues with your family; party organizer; travel planner, "rememberer" of most things you're likely to forget, etc.

Unfortunately, there is one role that is of great importance to you—and to her—that she usually has no role model for. That of lover. Because among women, there is still a shroud of shame that envelopes the topic of sex and intimacy. Mothers find it excruciatingly difficult to bring it up with their daughters, and even if they did, the conversation would most likely be about how men are only after one thing, followed by warnings to stay away from it altogether. Don't bother considering any advice from her father—who probably couldn't even bring up the topic of how to please a man with his own wife. Schools are hardly a source for information beyond the science—and prevention—of reproduction and STIs. And her girlfriends? It's rare for any woman to have a sexual health and best-practices authority as a friend.

Of course, a woman can choose to self-educate and read books or watch videos about it. But these would be limited in their coverage, with titles like *How to Drive Your Man Wild in Bed* or simply offering a range of sex positions and techniques any woman can try out with any man—even a stranger she just met at a bar. They're almost guaranteed to have a narrow definition of what a man wants. One thing's for sure, these "reference materials" won't be giving advice like, "S is for sex. So don't start the evening by treating your husband like your son, student, or servant."

Your partner needs to see herself as your lover; yet she may be clueless that even the sexiest lingerie won't work if she doesn't stand in your presence with the aura of a woman who desires you—for everything that you are. That making you feel seen, respected, and appreciated is what makes you want to come home and make love with her.

Honestly communicating about your emotional and sexual needs is key. Rules 2 and 3, to be discussed in later chapters, will give you a few clues on how to improve things in that department too.

Understanding the Many Sides of Her

This complexity that makes up your partner is why you need to get inside her mind now. Like that Rubik's cube, she's a puzzle Sherlock Holmes would love to solve. A mystery he'd enjoy unraveling. Not in a devious, cunning way, but through honest, open conversations.

Go much deeper than, "So what kind of music do you like?" just so you can surprise her with concert tickets to neutralize her emotional needs. Don't try to buy your way out of getting closer. She may seem happy and grateful for the moment, but in the long run, it doesn't work. You need to get closer by looking closer—into her mind, heart, and soul.

Be like Sherlock Holmes and ask questions that lead you to meaningful answers. Now that you know your mission, do you know hers? What does she value most in life? Has she figured it out? Is it compatible with yours?

You now know the value of self-love. Does she? Or is she using you as a crutch to love all the parts of her she couldn't? Does she think you're Mr. Right only because you complete the parts of her that she believes are still wrong? In much the same way that it's not a woman's job to fix the man she loves, no amount of romance from you can fix someone who was never whole.

If you come to a realization that she does indeed rely on you to compensate for her lack of self-love, it's also possible that this very "incompleteness" that she (subconsciously) feels is something you sensed too and could have been one reason you were drawn to her. Like everyone else, a man likes to feel needed and being involved with a woman who seems to be dependent on him could have its attraction. For one thing, it makes a man feel safe—that she would be less likely to leave or betray him. But problems begin once she senses your emotional distance. And you're bound to stay emotionally distant if you weren't invested in the *real* woman to begin with.

Ask questions. Observe. And learn.

To deepen your relationship, you need to ask the right questions and observe her in a variety of activities that would reveal the parts of her she's kept hidden for fear you wouldn't like the inner her (just like you may have hidden parts of yourself too). By keeping yourself emotionally unavailable, your commitment might be limited *to the state* of being in a relationship—and not to the woman herself.

It's unavoidable that some of you reading this might realize that you've settled. Meaning, not settled down with someone you truly cared for but settled for someone less than you had hoped for. It's possible that it's because, at the time, you didn't hold yourself in high regard, and you believed she was as good as it gets. Or maybe you had simply let the relationship happen because it filled in parts of the incomplete puzzle that was you—even though you knew she was just someone you liked but not really loved.

This works both ways, of course. Many women can settle too. But as time goes by, she can continue to grow in her self-worth and one day, she blinks and realizes she could do much better. You, on the other hand, could blink just in time to see her walking out the door.

That is one sad scenario. And that's what the three rules given in this book can help safeguard you against. If you dove into your relationship led by your gut or your groin without getting to know her that well, it's not too late. You can start asking questions now.

"Don't do it the way I would, though," Sherlock Holmes pipes in, seated on a tufted leather wing chair. "Not like some shrewd detective." He leans back and puts on a relaxed air. "Ask like a gentleman who'd like to get to know the lovely lady in front of him a little better."

Ask in a manner that will make the both of you fall deeper in love.

Count yourself fortunate if you'd gotten to know each other really well from the start, with both of you opening up to each other and allowing yourselves to be vulnerable. If in that climate of honesty, your bonds grew even tighter, then what you have now may well be a beautiful, profound relationship on a solid bedrock of friendship and emotional intimacy. If you are each other's best friend, many couples will envy y

"Ev

"or pe

never-

It's

stale b

know

years.

change

us are

keep yo

week.

differen

> *Think about yourself a year ago 3 years, 5 years Are you the same person, have your interests changed, had you discovered new things, made new friends. all of us are a work of art that's truly never completed*
>
> *5-19-2024*

And empathize with how she feels. Let her vent and just listen. Lend her your ear. In exchange, ask her to give you silence and space when it's your turn to mull over your bad day (if that's what you need). Don't try to "solve" her feelings; you just need to validate them. Fixing her feelings is not your purpose in her life. Instead, feel her feelings with her. She needs to know you're invested *in her*.

What does it mean "to validate" her feelings? If at the end of a long day, she gripes about a co-worker who's lazy and is the weakest link in the chain, even though your instinct urges you to tell her how to solve it, don't. Resist saying, "Why don't you just _____?" I know part of you will say what's the point of discussing a problem if you're not going to talk about a solution. Just don't. Instead, feel her feelings. Say something like, "Well, that would ruin my day too." Step into the pool of mud with her and let it cake around you. Don't suggest stepping out of the mud and hosing herself down with what you think is the best course of action. Just nod and let her pour it out. It's not for you to solve (unless she asks you to). Understand how your brains are wired. You deal with your feelings by growing silent and thinking things through; she deals with hers by talking about it and letting it out. That's how she sees things better. She's not holding her feelings out for you to fix them, burden, or blame you. Mainly, it's for her to get it off her chest and then she will love you more for seeing her side of things and just being there for her.

Take an interest in her interests and tell her about yours, so you keep getting to know each other again and again. Day after day.

Holmes rises from his seat and asks us to stuff our detective's caps into our Knapsack of Knowledge. He tells us that he's given us those to serve as a reminder of the things we've learned while in his company.

- Like a Rubik's cube, there are many fascinating sides to a woman. Some roles that she's comfortable with—such as that of mother, teacher, and boss—may feel uncomfortable when she goes into that role with you. Unless you really want her to, make sure you don't give her cues that tell her to treat you like her son, pupil, or orderly.

- There are things from her past that may be affecting how she relates to you. What did love look like to her in her youth? Most likely, the role of lover is not something she was taught.

- When you ask about her day and she starts to lament about her problems, don't try to solve them, unless she asks you to. Simply listen and validate her feelings. Let her know you understand and that you see things the way she sees them too. She doesn't expect you to "fix her feelings."

Holmes guides us towards the door and holds it open for us as he bids us farewell. "Remember," he says, tapping on the detective's cap on his head, "appreciate every facet of the wonderful woman you chose. Know who you love and why."

I nod back at him, grateful for his choice of words. Because the topic of "wonder-ful" women is exactly where I'm taking you next on our last stop in understanding Rule No. 1.

BE SUPERMAN TO YOUR WONDER WOMAN. YOU'RE BOTH HEROES WITH YOUR OWN BATTLES TO FIGHT.

RULE NO. 1: KNOW WHO YOU LOVE—AND WHY

Before I take you any further on this journey—where I'll be recruiting a couple of superheroes to help me illustrate my next point—let's take a moment to talk more about Rule No. 1: Know who you love—and why.

The answer to "why" may not be that hard for most people to figure out. It could be a nice character trait, how they make you feel, how they treat you. But what could be difficult to see is the reason why no matter how hard some couples try, there are conflicts that cannot seem to get resolved. This section explores a possible answer to, "Why not?"

Much of this book will be expounding on the differences between the physical, mental, and emotional makeup of the sexes. But it's highly likely those differences aren't the main or only reasons you and your lady don't see eye to eye on many things. One other key factor could be a possible clash in your attachment styles. So let's take a quick look at this major variable.

The Theory of Attachment

In case you're not familiar with the concept, attachment theory proposes that our early experiences with our caregivers have long-term effects that influence our emotions, defenses, behavior, and overall expectations in all our close relationships into adulthood (i.e. close friends, family, and intimate partners). These "paradigms" of bonding that we learn as children and carry into our adult relationships are what are referred to as attachment styles.

The theory of attachment was originally developed by psychoanalyst John Bowlby. It suggests that we're all born with a need to forge bonds with our parents or caregivers, so we'll have better chances of survival as infants, in case of external threats. The theory proposes that these early interactions get internalized by the child and turn into *paradigms* of expectations of care. Remember my question, "What did love look like when you were a child?" Well, these could turn into expectations of what we expect love to be like, and these expectations seem to stay in place into adulthood.

These are the things which the researchers took note of during the experiments: when the mother left her one-year-old son alone in a room with his toys, did the child become mildly distressed, inconsolable, or unruffled? And on the mother's return, did the child get easily soothed or did he continue to fret or was indifferent? It was initially proposed that the pattern of responses the child displayed were innate, but further research indicated that it may be reflective or a result of the caregiver's own attachment style. (In other words, the apple doesn't fall far from the tree.)

Bowlby's research, which began in the 1950s, focused on understanding the nature of the infant-caregiver relationship. There is now a growing body of research suggesting that adult romantic relationships do function in ways similar to infant-caregiver relationships. (Yes, how you were raised affects how you expect to be treated—or how you end up treating your partner—in an intimate relationship.) You can search online or read books for a deeper dive into the theory's history and further studies conducted by Ainsworth, Main, Bartholomew, Horowitz, Hazan, Shaver, Fraley, and many others—researchers whose findings have contributed to and continue to refine our understanding of the critical role these early relationships have in a person's healthy development, even influencing our intimate emotional relationships in adulthood. Tracking the depth and breadth of that knowledge is too much of a detour for us to take on this journey of ours, so I'll do my best to distill that wealth of information into a few pages for an easy-to-digest explanation relevant to romantic relationships.

These are the four recognized attachment styles, how the children exhibited them, and how they are reflected in adult attachments:

- **Secure**: Children show distress when separated from their mother but are easily soothed and regain their positive attitude quickly. Securely attached adults are comfortable with intimacy and have a healthy balance of dependence and independence in relationships.

- **Anxious/Preoccupied:** Children here show intense distress when their mother leaves but resist contact when the mother returns. Adults with this attachment style crave intimacy and can be overly demanding and dependent in relationships.

- **Dismissive/Avoidant:** Children show no outward signs of distress when separated from their mother and remain uninterested in their mother's return. Adults with this style display a strong sense of self-sufficiency, valuing their independence highly. They seem uninterested in close relationships to the point of appearing detached.

- **Fearful-Avoidant/Disorganized**: Children might be distressed to be left with an unfamiliar caregiver, but when the mother returns, will run to the unfamiliar person instead. As adults, they usually crave intimate relationships but are uncomfortable with closeness. They find it hard to trust others and are fearful of getting hurt, so they may end up sabotaging their own relationships.

What's important to note is that the theory does *not* assume or dictate that these paradigms or attachment styles persist without changing throughout a person's life. There are attachment theorists who have put forth a model that assumes existing paradigms are updated and eventually overwritten in light of new experiences one might have. So consider these attachment styles more like dimensions of anxiety and avoidance that continue to shift in varying degrees.

Imagine a line with arrows on both ends pointing left and right where you can indicate your level of anxiety about your feelings of security in your relationships—signifying low to high anxiety as you move from left to right. Then imagine another arrow pointing upwards and downwards, indicating your level of avoidance of others and your need to be close—signifying low to high avoidance as you move upwards. Plot your levels of anxiety and avoidance on those two dimensions, then superimpose these two arrows centered on a square, dividing the square into four quadrants. The intersection of where the plotted points on those two arrows are indicates the category you're in right now.

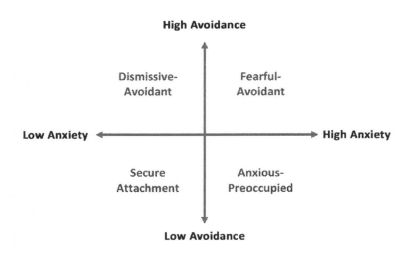

Based on the chart, those who are SECURE would have low anxiety, low avoidance. They hold a positive view of themselves and of others. Because of the consistent and responsive care they received as children, they feel comfortable relying on and getting close to others.

ANXIOUS/PREOCCUPIED individuals will have high anxiety, low avoidance. Due to inconsistent caregiving, they usually have low self-esteem but hold others in higher regard. This style is characterized by high emotional dependency, seeking intimacy and security from others, but finding it hard to trust. They worry about their partner's behavior and intentions, and they can be hyper-vigilant at spotting potential threats to their relationship.

The DISMISSIVE/AVOIDANT person would register low anxiety, high avoidance. They have a positive view of themselves, yet even as they view themselves as resilient, self-reliant, and independent, they hold a negative view of others and continue to have negative expectations because of the early unresponsive care they experienced. They tend to deny their need to connect emotionally, avoiding closeness, intimacy, and dependence on others.

Finally, those with FEARFUL-AVOIDANT/ DISORGANIZED attachment styles will have high anxiety, high avoidance. This developed when the child's caregivers became a source of intense fear, and they're still dealing with the long-term effects of this childhood trauma, neglect, or abuse. They usually have a negative view of themselves and of others. Because their caregivers became a source of both comfort and fear, it led to disorganized behavior. They desire close relationships yet fear vulnerability, and because of this internal conflict, they may behave unpredictably in relationships resulting in an approach-and-avoidance style of behavior.

After reading these broad descriptions, many people can immediately relate to one of the attachment styles or even categorize their intimate partner under one of them. Perhaps you can also tell how a clash in attachment styles can pose major challenges to a couple. If, let's say, you're dismissive/avoidant—which means you're highly independent and don't feel comfortable sharing your feelings—and you're in a romantic relationship with an anxious/preoccupied woman who needs constant check-ins, reassurances, and expressions of your love and fidelity ... I suppose you can complete the picture of how the anxious type could keep demanding something the other person is simply too avoidant to give.

To reiterate, where you plot yourself on the anxiety and avoidance scale can slide left or right and up or down in those dimensions, depending on your experiences and how you cope or learn from them.

So rather than placing yourself under one category permanently, think of it as two dimensions in which you may move with lesser or greater intensity, indicating what quadrant you're in at that particular stage in your life.

Overall, research findings indicate that secure adults tend to be more satisfied in their relationships compared to those with the other three attachment styles. Their relationships demonstrate greater longevity, trust, commitment, and interdependence. By interdependence, it means they continue to enjoy their independence while using their romantic partners as a secure base from which to explore the world.

If you're insecurely attached, your childhood traumas may be tough to get over on your own. It would be good to open up to a secure person who you feel safe with to guide you through your self-realizations. There have been situations when a dismissive/avoidant in a secure relationship slowly unlearned their dismissive behaviors, became more communicative of their emotional needs, and grew to be secure. Generally though, when it comes to the insecurely attached, the assumptions they make regarding their partners' actions during and after relational conflicts end up intensifying their insecurities. Healing your childhood wounds, therefore, and making the shift may be difficult or unlikely if you're both insecurely attached. Seeing a counselor or therapist would help make the process smoother.

That's something most of us didn't realize when growing up. We were going through our nights and days in robotic mode—living our lives based on programming we'd received as little children. If we're lucky, we've since come across new information that points out flaws in that programming, illuminating possible causes to hitches and glitches in our adult relationships.

What this new information gives us is the power to override.

Flick the switch inside you. All the books in all the libraries, and no number of hours with a therapist can amount to any change if *you* don't flick that switch yourself. The only things other people can provide you with are guidance and insights. It's only you who can flick that switch that will turn your life—and most valued relationships—towards where you want them to go.

My Own Shift in Attachment Styles

I love my mother dearly and believe she's one of the best mothers anyone could be blessed with. She did her utmost to attend to my needs and that of my four siblings, but with a family of that size, she needed to become a businesswoman to help supplement my father's income. Her business was home-based, so she was always around, but always extremely busy. So even though hers was the first face to greet me every morning in my early years, and the last to wish me goodnight, I spent most of my time alone with my books and toys and a sizable backyard where I could climb trees. Because I was a late addition to the family, my siblings were already of school age by the time I was born. So sometimes, my mother brought me to our neighbors' or close relatives' homes just so I could have playmates and wouldn't be alone.

If you were to plot me on that attachment chart, therefore, I would have had low anxiety, because I felt secure in my mother's love and concern for my well-being, but perhaps I'd be midway in terms of dismissiveness due to my not needing to get close to anyone, because I had learned to be at home with myself. I grew up happy even when alone.

After I became a parent, I opened up and became very emotionally available to my children. But when my marriage ended, I realized that the dismissive/avoidant part of me, though slight, had added to the emotional distance between me and my partner. Since then, I've been reaching out more to friends and family, sharing my feelings, allowing myself to be more vulnerable to others. And I must say, it feels good.

Later in the book, when we get to Rule No. 3, I'll be sharing insights on how you, too, can feel your feelings and soften them up. For now, let's stay here with Rule No. 1, and talk about why you need to be a Superman to your Wonder Woman.

A Strong Man and a Strong Woman

We climb to the top of a dry and dusty mesa—a rocky, flat-topped hill with a good view of the road ahead and behind us. Wonder Woman bursts out of the clear blue sky and makes a superhero landing with a heart-stopping thud on the ground, shattering the slab of rock underneath her. We're suddenly covered in dust from head to toe, but we don't mind. We don't care. Damn. It's dust stirred up by Wonder Woman!

The sun's brightness flickers for a moment as Superman swoops by overhead.

"Holy crap," you say. "If he lands the same way, this whole mountain could crack in two."

Superman pauses midflight and hovers at the edge of the hill we're on. We all gawp at him as he touches down gently on a slate of rock, back straight, shoulders squared, his cape flapping in the wind.

"Why the quiet entrance?" Wonder Woman asks as his feet touch the earth.

Superman glances at you. "I heard not everyone here is a fan of hard landings."

You gulp, and the sound seems to reverberate around the canyon.

"That's all right," Superman says with a smile. "Neither am I."

For a few seconds, we all just stand in quiet awe, staring at the two larger-than-life crusaders, and try to pick our jaws up off the dusty ground.

Wonder Woman glances around at us. "Would you be more at ease if we talked with you as Clark Kent and Diane Lane instead?"

"No, this is perfect," I say, stepping forward. "Because I needed you here as superheroes to help me out with this topic." I point upwards. "It's over there."

Everyone looks up at the sky.

"No, not there," I say. "A few pages back, actually."

I break the fourth wall on paper, and their brows knot as they stare at me.

"It's at the top of this section of the book." I thrust my thumb upwards. "Remember the title of this part? It says, 'Be a Superman to your Wonder Woman.' I didn't say *versus* Wonder Woman, because I wanted to draw attention to how two strong people should be able to become a happy couple and not end up in a so-called 'battle of the sexes.'"

You shake your head. "But they aren't together. He's with Lois Lane and she's in love with Steve Trevor."

"My point exactly." I look at the power couple. "Why is that?"

Superman cocks a brow at me. "Why aren't we together?"

I nod.

The two exchange glances, and Superman shrugs his broad shoulders. "Ask the comic book writers. They gave it a shot in the DC Comics universe, but it didn't last."

"Really?" you ask, your curiosity piqued. "What happened?"

"The writers made me lose my powers," Superman says, "and I ended up dying."

Wonder Woman, grim-faced, crosses her arms. "And that left me right back where I started. Strong, super, and single."

"Just like with Steve Trevor." I sigh and shake my head. "Why don't we have superhero stories that show us a strong man living happily ever after with a strong woman?" (I'm discounting Pixar's *The Incredibles* because that celebrates family more than romance.)

"I think it's because fiction also needs inspiration from real life." Superman gazes out at the horizon using his telescopic vision. "And it's not that easy to find."

Life Beyond Lois Lane and Mary Jane

A lot of men like to picture themselves as superheroes out to impress the Lois Lanes and Mary Janes—ordinary mortal females who need to be saved or seem in some way "less" than they are. But these days, women are very much superheroes in their own fields and at the end of the day, they come home just as battered and bruised as you with their own tales of adventure.

But that's not to say that all women have grown to have this mindset. There will still be those far more comfortable with the traditional feminine role of homemaker with her husband as the breadwinner. If that's the situation you're in or that's the kind of dynamic you prefer, then this section may not seem relevant to you, although I encourage you to read it for the sake of getting a new perspective on these gender-role changes happening globally. It would be unfortunate for you to find out too late if your partner is only giving up her dreams because she fears she would lose you or would not be fulfilling her expected role if she didn't. She might have come across certain blogs and videos in social media wherein "macho men" influencers describe their ideal woman as someone submissive, attentive to his needs, feminine, and subservient to his wishes. I'm afraid this could cause confusion in some women who may not be getting better guidance in their personal lives.

If she's happy to be in that traditional role and that's truly how she's envisioned her future life as a wife and that matches your life's vision too, then you've found your match.

For all other men who feel that relationships have grown more challenging because of female empowerment and the uncertainty of where the line is that turns masculinity toxic, then I hope these next few paragraphs help give some clarity.

Women Then and Now

There was a time when all a woman needed to do to get a nod from society was find a husband and raise a family. She wasn't expected to get a job. And if she did, it was all right if she remained at the bottom rung—like a factory worker who never got to be the supervisor. If anything, success and a strong financial position were more like "options" she pursued for her own gratification and were unnecessary because, tradition says, the men already had that covered. Her success in her career, therefore, was considered redundant among married couples.

It's having this old-world mentality that deprives many men today the chance to embrace relationships with sparklingly intelligent, independent-minded women who have achieved or are pursuing their own level of success. It's a shame that men steer clear of them, as proven by research in this area.[16] When asked, hypothetically, if the men would be interested in dating strong, smart, successful women, nearly 90%

said yes. But presented with the reality of meeting her, the men backed away, particularly if the woman had performed better than him in an intelligence test. If the woman was already in the same room, he would place his chair farther away from her but position it closer if he's told that she had scored lower than him in the test. As an abstract concept, a smart, independent, successful woman is deemed highly desirable—but not when she turns into a real figure at arm's reach. (Interestingly, even in the online gaming community, research shows that men try much harder to win when they perceive their opponent to be a woman.)[17]

More and more women are opting to stay single. As of 2021, a record-breaking 52% of women in America are unmarried or separated. Between 2002 and 2018 in the UK, the percentage of women in their 40s who've never married doubled in those fifteen years. In India, there are currently more single women than at any other time, while East Asian countries have also seen a significant rise in the number of single households, driven by the individual's decision to stay unmarried.

One reason could simply be that being single and childless no longer carries the stigma it used to. Women are marrying later in life or choosing not to remarry after a divorce with freedom as their priority. The terms "old maid" and "spinster" are already considered politically incorrect, and words such as happy and single can now belong in the same sentence.

Another perspective is that modern women are probably wondering what they need a husband for. Women graduating from college now outnumber men, and the number of women in managerial positions continues to climb, giving them financial independence that was once unthought of. The police and firefighters are everywhere, one text or call away, giving a sense of security women of yesteryears didn't have. And unlike before, when virginity was something saved for the honeymoon, women can now choose to treat sex as casually as men do. They buy sex toys and are far less inhibited in pleasuring themselves. They can even opt to have children without a man and just head to the nearest sperm bank.

Taking a look at the data, men need to pause and think seriously. The vast majority of divorces are initiated by women, 63% in the UK, about 80% in the US, and 74% in China. And as for women who've never been married, more are choosing to stay single worldwide as well. Wonderful women out there are wondering about the value of their romantic relationships with men.

Why Men Steer Clear of Wonder Woman

The love story between Steve Trevor and Wonder Woman is a rarity in the world of superheroes. For those unfamiliar with the DC universe, Steve is a military officer with no supernatural powers or weapons and was the first man the immortal Amazon princess ever laid eyes on and who eventually won her heart. Their story is genuinely moving and leaves you feeling good about how they balance their differences, despite him being an ordinary human—albeit a noble, brave, and handsome one. What makes them stand out as a couple is that it is the female with the superpowers while the man remains undaunted and remains by her side, supportive and responsive to her needs.

Such a pairing need not stay stuck in the world of fantasy and fiction. Their counterparts, brought down to mortal Earth, would be a highly successful, desirable woman married to a man who has risen to a level just high enough to be worthy of her respect, love, and admiration which she expresses and demonstrates to him every single day.

Admittedly though, that's a pairing that's relatively simple on paper but difficult to come by in real life.

There are many women today who could end up scoring higher than you on intelligence tests and are capable of becoming equal or better leaders and managers. They could also look hot, earn more than you, and be in their element at social gatherings. Alpha women are everywhere. And if we're to go by the research, men are steering clear of them.

Why? Quite likely, it's because most people still haven't quite let go of the way things were: The male-female dynamic of "Me Tarzan, You Jane," the man being the strong and dominant protector and the female being the damsel in distress. Things began to change during World War II, when women left their homes and went to work to take the place of droves of men who'd gone off to defend the motherland. When the world quieted down and the gunpowder settled, mothers continued to raise their sons like future soldiers, but the daughters were now being told they could be what they wanted to be.

The problem is that this change happened under the radar. It was not preached in pulpits, taught in schools, or broadcast in the media. Without fanfare, more and more young girls grew up to become mothers who entered and thrived in the work force, changing the norm in most homes. Dad was no longer Tarzan who swung home to a plain Jane homemaker. Mom was now out all day in the concrete jungle too. But the sons—who include you—continued to be painted a picture of Dad being the provider who came home to Mom who, despite having spent the day at work as well, prepared dinner, helped the kids with their homework, and was in-charge of keeping the home spic and span. This means there was a mismatch between the mental picture of a homebound mother and the reality of a working mom, compounded by a tug of war between how men wanted things to remain and how women wanted things to change.

This is the line where masculinity can turn toxic. When a man's attitude towards a woman is based on a perception that she is emotionally or intellectually inferior to him, or physically "at his disposal." When he conveys that her personal achievements and success are of no value to him, and what makes him value her is simply having her support and respect him, this attitude is something she can discern. As such, it becomes a rejection of her dreams and a denial of her worth. Surprisingly, this sentiment among women isn't all that modern. My mother was born in 1926, and even she resented my father when he implied that he didn't value her college education and what mattered was that she was a good wife. So take this word of caution. Some of you might think you're in a relationship with a "traditional gal" who likes it the way things were. But no matter what social class or level of education, I've seen it happen. Even among the poorest of the poor, when the woman feels her man looks down on her for simply being a woman, she wants out of there.

Things go overboard, however, when holding the door open for a woman or offering to pay for dinner are translated into statements to mean she's weak or unable to provide for herself. These, to me, are gracious acts of chivalry that I believe should be allowed to live on. Just as a female boss would still make a cup of coffee for her husband or a female bodybuilder would still ask her boyfriend to open a jar of mayonnaise for her, certain everyday acts of kindness are no longer signs of subservience or helplessness but have turned into gestures of courtesy, affection, and appreciation.

Women don't need to be weak or dependent to need or want a man in her life. Not believing or comprehending this could be why a man might feel uneasy and sometimes downright scared of being in a relationship with a woman he deems "out of his league." Going back to this book's premise, we have no famous role models for such a paradigm besides Steve Trevor and Wonder Woman. So let's work with what we have and cut through all the thorny issues, reducing things to one simple superhero point.

What's the major reason the relationship between Steve Trevor and Wonder Woman works? Steve is responsible, supportive, and openly loving. For her part, she doesn't treat him like her son, pupil, or subordinate. And that's what makes a relationship with Wonder Woman so wonderful. Man and woman accord each other all the respect and admiration each deserves, so both feel loved, appreciated, and irreplaceable. Regardless of who was stronger, smarter, or more "super" than the other, what mattered was that they made each other feel good.

Which is why, if you didn't take the previous section to heart—about being Sherlock Holmes knowing the woman you love—I suggest you go back and do so now. Because if you're going through the trouble of reading this book and applying its principles, you should ask yourself first: Are you with the right woman? If so, then your relationship is worth your superhero effort to make it work—if you're with an emotionally secure woman whose values align with yours, accepts you for who you are, and is with you for the right reasons.

Why Wonder Woman Needs Superman

We're back on the rocky and dusty mesa. The sun is hanging low in the sky and the two superheroes are looking down at the road stretching ahead of us.

"You have quite a way to go on this hero's journey," Superman says.

"But it will be worth it," Wonder Woman says.

"Could I ask you something?" you say, taking a step forward. "What do you think about men who've 'met their match'—like a Superman meeting his Wonder Woman—and falling for her? Do you think this can work in real life?"

"I'd like to think that that's what most couples are aiming for today," Wonder Woman answers with a smile. "Two remarkable individuals, successful in their own fields, who have found someone who feels like home."

You turn to me. "What do you think? Can it work?"

Everyone else looks at me too.

I clear my throat. "It's possible that it's more common in reality than it is in fiction. Because when it comes to a superhero and a superheroine nurturing a long-term romantic relationship—in the world of comics, we have yet to see one that works. They usually need to choose between their superhero lives and each other—or one of them dies."

Superman snorts. "You can say that again."

I glance at the formidable female standing next to him. It must be a puzzle in men's heads—and comic book writers. Why would Wonder Woman need any man at all? She's a mighty warrior princess who needs no protector. Wouldn't he just add to her immense load of things to look after already? She's an immortal demigoddess who needs no provider. And she's drop-dead gorgeous who can get any man she wants.

And let's not forget the research. Most men will steer clear of her because of her brains and everything previously mentioned above. Which is why the stereotypical male superhero falls for Lois Lanes and Mary Janes. Smart and sassy women but mere mortals, nonetheless. They're the ones the mighty men choose to come home to.

And therein lies your answer. Why would Wonder Woman need any man at all? It's for the same reason male superheroes need any woman. After a day of flying and swooping and swinging around, every person—man or woman, super or not—needs a soft place to land. And no matter how many people out there may look up to and rely on us, when we come home and the sun goes down and everything becomes quiet, we just want to look in someone else's eyes and find peace.

We want somebody we don't have to compete with. Someone who won't judge us or make us feel small. Someone we can hold in our arms and in whose company we can relax and be vulnerable. It's a mistake to think that such a woman can only be someone who embodies the fragile female of the past.

That's why men who are hanging on to the old-world setup where women stayed in the kitchen, let the man wear the trousers, and just kept her apron on are depriving themselves of a superb experience. That of lying next to a woman who could be his trusted warrior against daily battles, a cunning partner in solving life's troubles, and his amazing, loving goddess in bed.

Today's woman can buy necessities and luxuries for herself. Though she may prefer not to, she's capable of raising the kids on her own. She has her own passions, successes, and her own mission in life. And if her man fails to recognize that and still sees her as much like his grandmother was to his granddad, then he stands to lose her.

It is unfortunate if you believe her success is unimportant and doesn't interest you. That if she wants to talk about her day and her frustrations, then she should call a girlfriend instead of telling you. That her thinking about everything everywhere all at once except sex is a huge turnoff.

Money can get you a maid, a hooker, a therapist, and a nanny. If all you want is someone to take care of your needs without you having to reciprocate, then use your money. If all you want is to have fun and not bother with feelings, hopes, and dreams, then use the time to have a drink with your buddies. Or get yourself a pet.

A Soft Place to Land

We've stayed long enough on Rule No. 1—where you got to know yourself a little better as well as your partner by asking her the right questions. You now also have a better understanding of attachment styles and how the modern woman needs a modern man in vastly different ways than how her grandmother needed her grandfather. Grandma needed grandpa to survive. Your partner needs you to feel seen, heard, and loved.

It's time to set off for Rule No. 2.

Before we head down the hill, Wonder Woman looks at you with deep-set eyes that reveal how she's come to be known as the champion of empathy.

"When someone falls in love," she says, "no matter how strong they are, they can't bear to lose that person. They'd be left with an empty space that no one else can fill. That space is in her arms, her mind, and in her heart. She set aside that space just for you."

Superman nods. "Be a Brave Heart," he says, "and allow yourself to get close enough to someone until she makes you feel weak enough to need her. Then let her know—in every possible way—how much she means to you. Give her a soft place to land."

Wonder Woman glances at the slab of rock she'd shattered when she first arrived. "I suggest you all take a shard of that rock along with you, as a reminder of the lessons learned today."

We smile with gratitude and wave as the two superheroes fly off and leave us to complete our journey.

I bend down and pick up a piece of rock from the ground for my Knapsack of Knowledge. "You know who you love—and why. And now, you know that allowing yourself to be vulnerable is part of being the Superman that your Wonder Woman needs."

If you want to be a man who can conquer the strongest, smartest, sexiest woman in your life—so *you* can always have that soft place to land—then read the next section and learn how to give her exactly that.

4

Rule No. 2: Do Things that Show Her You Love Her

This seems like a no-brainer, but something as overt as an action can still get lost in translation. It's surprising how many women end up frustrated because how her partner demonstrates his love doesn't match with her definition.

Earlier, I'd stated that an overwhelming majority of divorces are initiated by the woman. I also gave statistics showing that an increasing number of women are choosing to stay single. What was the major reason that was cited? It's that men still act like they're Superman married to a Lois Lane who's willing to do all the housework while he gets to bask in the sun and regenerate his powers. Of course, the research doesn't say it that way, but that's what it boils down to. Many men still behave in ways that don't acknowledge how the women they're with are as heroic as they are, so the man still goes about his days pouring superhuman effort into his job and assumes she's happy and content taking care of the house he comes home to.

I honestly don't think men mean to be stubborn about changing. My educated guess is that it's unclear to most men what's expected of them, because they hadn't been taught how a wife wants and needs to be treated by the people he considered the primary authorities on the topic: His parents.

Most mothers are still raising their sons the way their fathers had been raised—to be a soldier, a hunter, or a superhero—taught to be a stranger to his own feelings. And a son looks to his father for how to treat his wife, and what he learns is usually just a minor revision of how his grandfather had treated his wife. The mother still shows her son how it's all in a day's work for a wife to juggle a career with the responsibilities of caring for her home, husband, and children. The father still shows his son how he has the right to stay busy and emotionally distant as he provides for his family. Rarely, if ever, will the son hear any snippets of wisdom from his mother saying, "This is how a woman wants to be loved. Beyond giving her roses and vacations. Beyond the fancy dinner dates. This is how a man keeps a woman's heart beating for him till death do us part." Of course, she need not sound as syrupy as that—but she does need to give her son an idea of what sweet love between husband and wife means.

Sadly, most of the time, what a son sees and learns is that the father is the man of the house until his mother grows tired and one day walks out of that house. But nobody explains why it happened. All they learn is that love doesn't last. Fighting is inevitable. And that it wasn't the son's or any of the children's fault. If the parents never separated, it's a lucky boy who has memories of a warm and loving couple devoted to each other's happiness as they were raising him. (Of course, there will always be exceptions and varying scenarios. I, for one, never saw my parents fight until after they were separated by the time all the children had grown up—an example which I'd unwittingly modeled my own marriage after.)

And so the son, now a grown man, walks out into the world, with memories of his parents fighting or just tolerating each other but still holding on to a wish to have his own family someday. So he braces for the worst, hopes for the best, goes out and enters the dating game, polishing (a.k.a. faking) his profile, and hoping for someone to fall for him.

But maybe, just maybe, you can put a stop to this paralyzing mess. Seeing things from a new perspective, you can be an agent of change. Read on and find some answers as to why many marriages fail and what you can do to keep it from happening to yours.

Once again, it takes two to tango—as a reminder that I'm not putting the onus of making relationships work on men alone or that it's the men's fault that women can feel let down. That was the entire point of Rule No. 1 of knowing who you love and why. There are definitely times when a man ends up with a woman who's simply not right for him. Perhaps she, or he, or both of them have negative personality traits or unresolved childhood traumas that have more difficult solutions and are beyond what this book alone can do anything about.

This chapter will have three subsections that will draw inspiration from a new set of fictional characters:

- James Bond – with a new perspective on being the object of your affection

- Q – with advice on the best aphrodisiac

- Prince Charming – with a new definition of courtship

We'll then cap it all off with our buried treasure, hoping to find the answer to, "What does a woman want?"

BE BETTER THAN JAMES BOND. DON'T GET A BOND GIRL. BOND WITH YOUR GIRL.

RULE NO. 2: DO THINGS THAT SHOW HER YOU LOVE HER

We're in a casino in the middle of the desert. There aren't many people around, but the place is brightly lit by lavish chandeliers that showcase the posh interior and bold colors of the carpet. We're here to observe—not exactly to meet—James Bond, a timeless icon of masculinity whose 007 station in life seems to be all he needs to have it all. It's what gives him his fancy gadgets, luxurious lifestyle, and a suave persona.

Bond appears at the doorway with a bombshell on his arm, and it's as if spotlights have been turned on even though the room's brightness hasn't changed. He stands tall, dapper, and dashing. She's also tall and simply drop-dead gorgeous.

"How does he always get them?" one of us asks a little too loudly.

Bond acts as if he hasn't heard and moves closer to our table. "One thing's for sure—" He tugs on the cuff of his sleeve with diamond-encrusted cuff links. "I've never had to wear my heart on my sleeve." He glances at the voluptuously dressed woman whose arm is wrapped around that tuxedo sleeve.

She bats her thick lashes and looks up at him. "That's not how it works in real life, James," she says in a sultry voice. "At least, not anymore." She lets go of his arm and sashays her way to an empty cocktail table and slinks onto a seat.

Bond follows her—but only with his gaze, and only for a moment. Then he turns and strides towards the bar, away from her.

"I know. Shaken, not stirred," the bartender says, preparing Bond's drink even before he gets there.

"Not yet," Bond says. "I'm working." He orders a drink for the lady and heads off somewhere in the back of the casino and disappears.

To this day, if any other man had made an entrance like James Bond's—with a gorgeous woman on his arm—it still comes with the promise that, in that moment, his status instantly goes up within that group. But one has to keep in mind, it's great to feel proud about being in love with a beautiful woman, and it's another thing entirely when all you're proud of is that she's in love with you.

Bond may have turned his back on his date, but the lady has a point. With women asking for the overwhelming majority of divorces all over the world, there's good reason to believe the modern woman is not sticking around for a man who treats her like a mere accessory.

The original Bond Girls are among the classic examples of women being objectified, that is, being treated solely as an object of sexual desire. But what isn't clear to most men is that it's not the only way a woman can feel like she's being treated like an object. Even when a man swears to have a deep affection for the woman in his life and has no desire to offend her, he could still end up guilty of objectifying her in other ways.

That is the core of Rule No. 2: Do things that show her you love her. You may be thinking, "But I'm doing all of this for her! Isn't it obvious?"

You might be surprised. So I'll be giving a few examples to illustrate my point.

I apologize in advance if the following analogies end up hitting some sore spots. But I needed to use these "objects" to illustrate how a man's normal behavior can seem callous to a woman, even though the man is minding his own business or is behaving so in good faith to avoid ruffling her feathers or getting on her nerves.

So what are the different ways that a man can make his woman feel objectified?

A Box to Tick

For starters, she could feel like a ticked box on a checklist. Do you spend most of your time at home attending to chores, your own interests, or with your gadgets? Aside from sex, are there any meaningful things you would do *only for her* and with her—things you wouldn't do if she weren't in your life? You might take her out for dinner now and then, say "Love you" when the feeling strikes, and buy her some things every so often. But if your time alone together is relegated to shallow exchanges about household tasks, work, and the kids, she could see you as only investing the bare minimum, and the relationship ends up feeling like a box you just had to tick so you can call your life complete. Man cannot live on bread alone, whereas a woman cannot love on breadcrumbs alone.

A Trophy

Do you flaunt photos of her on social media and make sure to let others know how much you pamper her? Are you proud about having such a woman to call your own? That's great. But beyond that, how special do you make her feel when you're apart or when you're alone together? If not much goes on elsewhere, she could end up feeling like a trophy on a shelf that only gets polished now and then to make sure her feelings for you don't tarnish.

An Automobile

After investing so much of yourself in "acquiring" her, did you have a shift in attitude that made her feel like a car that you drove home and parked in a garage in the back of your head? In the meantime, do you go about your life, business as usual, simply revving her up now and then to keep things well-maintained? It does keep things simple, just having the car purring along, as long as you heed the warning lights on the dash. But to her, it could seem like you only pay her enough attention after every 5,000 miles—a kind of preventive maintenance against divorce.

(On a related note, some women might think that moving in together is like a test drive before marriage. Whereas for the man, it could simply mean ... moving in together, with marriage nowhere on the road ahead.)

Man's Best Friend

Not quite an "object," but even the most beloved canine companion cannot be likened to a spouse. And yet men who look for Bond Girls, particularly men with a "macho mentality," want someone they can proudly parade in front of others. Someone who joyfully greets him when he comes home, does what he says with no objections, then just lets him do his own thing when he's at home. When the man wants to play, man's best friend is expected to be eager to please. And all he needs to do is take her out once in a while, spend on her creature comforts, and give her a nice house to live in. "Good girl!"

Fish in the Water

Again, not quite an "object," but there is a common saying that when one is looking for a mate, there's lots of fish in the sea. So what does a man do? Bait them—with all the things he's heard that women want. The attention, the unforgettable dates, and yeah, even the mushy symbols of thoughtfulness and romance. And then, one of them falls for him—hook, line, and sinker. He hauls her out of the ocean and keeps her well-fed and well cared for in the aquarium of his life. And now she spends her days, floating in her new existence, wondering, "What happened to all that wonderfully delicious bait?"

A Wallet in the Back Pocket

Another way a woman can end up feeling like an object is when the relationship is treated like a wallet. And it has nothing to do with money. At the start of a relationship, you fill it up with wads and wads of attention and affection. Lots of precious time and whispered sweet nothings folded into a tight, secure bundle. Now, think of how you slip your wallet into your back pocket in the morning and sort of forget about it for the rest of the day. And you feel secure knowing that it's there and you only reach for it when you need it. That's how a man could treat his romantic relationship after some time—when his woman turns into a comforting presence in his back pocket. Out of sight, out of mind. But within easy reach and ready for him whenever he needs it.

Why Do Men "Objectify" Without Meaning To?

A man may have absolutely no intention of hurting his partner's feelings, and the last thing he wants to do is upset her. Unfortunately, even when the only thing he wants to do is keep the peace, his default means of keeping the peace is akin to keeping his distance. The effect? She ends up feeling like an object.

The old warning that was repeatedly given to your partner when she was a young girl—that men are after only one thing—still plays in her mind. And if she feels ignored or neglected or treated like an object, she will sense that shift in your demeanor when you suddenly turn on the killer charisma, or when you unexpectedly offer to help her with something, or you pay attention to what she's saying over dinner. Especially when it happens just a few minutes before you enter the bedroom. She will tense up inside, thinking "he's only after one thing." And if you've been focusing on work or had been keeping your distance before then, it could have caused her to build up some resentment against you. So you can't expect to pull her out of your back pocket and find a wad of eagerness waiting to unfold for you.

Bond Better than James Bond

Cyndi Lauper once sang, "Girls just wanna have fun." Perhaps during the dating stage, yes, but once they're in a relationship, many men would disagree with Cyndi's lyrics. Men end up steering clear of the girl when all the non-fun stuff starts building up. The complaints, criticism, rejection, drama, and a host of other negative triggers.

"Why can't we just have fun?" a friend lamented to me after he broke up with his live-in girlfriend. "Why did she have to bring all those emotions into the picture?"

I glanced down at the favorite of his two bulldogs lying next to his feet. "If all you want is companionship, doesn't he have all that covered?" I gestured to his pet.

My friend ignored me and shook his head. "We used to laugh a lot together. I just want fun! We used to just drink, laugh, and have fun."

I nodded. "You can get that with all the guys, can't you?" I was doing to him what I did to my male advertising students when I wanted them to figure out why a man would want to "import" a woman onto his all-male planet.

My friend stared at me as it slowly dawned on him that to let a woman into his life, he also needed to let emotions in—something he was raised to ignore by parents who were very "methodical" – that was the word he'd used to describe their parenting style. It drained him, the process of feeling. He didn't care about recognizing his wide range of emotions and naming them and learning to express them. He felt safe in the way his methodical world worked.

After that talk, he decided he was content with the life he had with his dogs and joked that he should just buy himself a camper and a sailboat and spend the rest of his life alone but happy. A joke, I believe, that really held a grain of truth.

If you're like him, someone who feels that opening up your heart to someone would suck the life out of you and take away the fun out of a relationship, you may be looking for a pet, a car, a trophy, a wad of security in your back pocket, or just simply another box to tick. But if you insist you want a woman in your life while still keeping her at a distance from your emotions, then you may be looking for a Bond

Girl. An object to fulfill your desires and who won't require much in return—except maybe your money (because just like James Bond, you know that diamonds are forever.)

The low drone of men talking drifts towards our table, and we realize, without us noticing exactly when, that Bond had returned. He's at the bar, downing the last of his martini cocktail. His cuff links glint as he checks the time on his Omega Seamaster. The lady, still seated alone at the cocktail table, notices his movement and sighs.

"Do you have somewhere to go?" she asks.

"Always," Bond replies.

He pays the bartender then goes over to her and holds out his hand … which she takes as she slides off her seat. She curls her hand around his arm and they walk out together, the same way they'd entered. Looking like a perfect couple for others to admire.

Our group exchanges glances after having observed what took place: How everything could look impeccable on the outside but feel sad and empty on the inside.

Knowing what you know now, of how staying distant and distracted can leave your woman feeling alone, can you imagine yourself out there working, fulfilling your mission, and fighting your fights—then you use the pause in the middle of gunfire to text her, "This is all for you." And mean it? Hats off to you! James Bond would rather get shot than do that. But you're better than him.

If you look forward to coming home to a loving woman at the end of every day, and despite being tired, you want to invest in quality time with her so you can *bond*—then keep reading.

BE HER JARVIS, Q, OR ALFRED. SHOW HER YOU HAVE HER BACK.

RULE NO. 2: DO THINGS THAT SHOW HER YOU LOVE HER

We step out of the casino and into the desert, just in time to catch the taillights of Bond's sports coupe disappearing into the night. Standing at the curb is Q, Quartermaster of MI6's research and development division. He's the one who's arranged for us to be allowed here tonight, the one who's provided everything Bond needs for his assignment, and who is now making sure we make it safely out of the desert in the dead of night.

He turns to us and asks, "Do you have a ride? I can provide you whatever it is you need."

I glance at the stretch of road barely lit by moonlight. "As much as we'd appreciate it, we're on a hero's journey. And it's not like racing out of here in sports cars is part of the quest." I chuckle.

Q nods. "I understand."

I reach out to shake his hand. "Thank you for your hard work and for thinking of our needs."

"I can provide you limousines instead," Q says, shaking my hand.

"No," I say. "I must decline."

"What?!" Everyone in our group objects.

"Why can't we take a limo?" you ask.

"Because *not* taking the easy way out is the lesson of this next leg of the journey. You've learned something from James Bond. Now it's time to learn from Q."

Q cocks his head. "I'm assuming you're talking about the hard work I put in to ensure the success of each assignment?"

"Yes," I nod, "precisely that."

The Little-known Aphrodisiac

It's second nature for a man to picture himself the superhero in the movie in his mind, and I have yet to meet a man who casts himself as the helper behind the scenes. Jarvis to Iron Man. Alfred to Batman. Q to James Bond. The reason I chose these characters for this section is to put the spotlight on how important it is for men to also play this role in their relationships.

Why does it matter? It's the little-known aphrodisiac that even women are often not aware of. Having a partner that helps take her mind off the many things she needs to get done helps her get in the mood phenomenally well.

For women who aren't interested in sex or have a difficult time achieving orgasm, one of the first things a sex therapist will talk about are the "brakes" and "accelerators" to her arousal. Different therapists may give each of these a different label, but in essence, brakes are those things that get in the way of her mind allowing herself to let go. One major brake is her inability to stop thinking of everything still on her to-do list.

Men are wired to focus on one thing at a time. It's a fundamental asset to being a good hunter. You tune out everything else and you focus on what's right in front of you and what needs to get done right now. So when you're at work, you think of work. When you're watching basketball, you think of basketball. When you're out drinking with your buddies, you think of what you're talking about while drinking with your buddies.

A woman who's at work will be thinking of her kids, what her husband might want for dinner, what's inside her pantry, and that she needs to call her mother before lunch to remind her about the new meds the doctor told her to start taking—and yes, of course, work. I don't think I need to illustrate what else might be on her mind when she's at the supermarket, doing yoga, watering the potted plants, or while driving to your kid's soccer practice. When night falls, after you and the family have had dinner, you watch a game on TV with a bottle of beer then decide to call it a night. You enter the bedroom and your wife is in bed with her iPad. You lock the door and cozy up to her and—if we're to go by numerous survey results— you'll be devoting about five to ten minutes to foreplay, and the entire act of lovemaking should be done in about 15 to 20 minutes, all in all.

That's assuming, of course, she agrees to it right away. But chances are, she won't be in the mood. She was on her iPad hoping to unwind because she's still stressed from her day. There's still laundry in the dryer, the cat litter box needs to be cleaned, and she plans to wake up early to dye her hair. So she looks at you with a harassed look on her face and grimaces as if to say, "I'm kind of tired, but if you insist, okay, fine." She doesn't say that, but she doesn't have to. The look on her face tells you it's another rejection. So you sigh as you slide quietly under the sheets and kiss her goodnight.

The Orgasmic Female Brain

Why does she do that? You wonder if she's deliberately sabotaging your sex life.

You wouldn't think that if you understood how much the female brain needs to let go to maximize her sexual experience. There is research conducted by Janniko Georgiadis and colleagues, scientists at the University of Groningen in the Netherlands, which indicates how parts of the brain that govern fear and anxiety are switched off when a woman is having her orgasm. This study, which mapped brain function during orgasm, revealed that areas of the brain that govern emotional control are also heavily deactivated as a woman climaxes. (For this study, the female volunteers were injected with a dye and laid on a scanning machine bed that revealed the switching off in certain areas of the brain. There is another research study though using fMRI that showed extensive cortical, subcortical, and brainstem regions peaking at orgasm and no evidence of deactivation of brain regions leading up to or during orgasm. Quite the opposite, this latter study sounds like the female brain is almost completely taken over when she climaxes. But this fMRI study had each volunteer's head constrained by a custom-fitted thermoplastic whole-head and neck brace stabilizer. So it makes me wonder how this methodology could have let each participant surrender completely to the pleasurable sensations to allow regions of her brain to deactivate with her head and neck clamped rigidly into place!)

Much of the research on what happens in the brains of men and women are often conflicting, perhaps this is also due to the variation in methodologies employed. But put simply, what they collectively show is that the brain needs to cooperate to get an orgasm to happen—as opposed to your heart that can keep on beating whether or not it's connected to your brain. So whether reaching orgasm requires the recruitment of most sections of the brain or their deactivation, it's not something the brain would be willing to do if the woman in charge is still thinking about everything everywhere all at once. Hunters are wired to home in on the kill at the crack of a twig; the gatherers, on the other hand, couldn't help but keep listening for twigs cracking in case the kids are wandering around, the dog hasn't been fed, or if her husband has left the fire burning outside.

And that's how being more like Q will help with your sex life. By doing things to eliminate some of her many concerns, you help get rid of the mental brakes that keep her from being in the moment with you. In short, make sure her mind is cleared of worries that will block her willingness to welcome pleasure.

You're probably wondering why this is an issue now whereas men in the past were oblivious to that list she has in her head when in the bedroom. The truth is, women have been faking orgasms for centuries, possibly millennia, and the women stayed in their marriages, nonetheless. But today's divorce statistics are showing that this list in her head needs minding from her partner too. Happy marriages are real-life partnerships, not mere contracts of union anymore.

[Allow me to take you aside for a moment for an off-road discussion about the "Invisible Load" that are crystal clear in women's minds but often imperceptible to many men's eyes. On top of the visible house chores you may be helping with, there's the mental load of planning, coordinating, and checking up on the day-to-day activities of the adults, kids, and other living things in the household, keeping track of what food is in the house, clothes, toys, bills, birthdays and other special occasions and gifts to give, visits to the doctor, dentist, vet, dealing with tantrums, schoolwork, sickness, or demotivated kids. And don't forget the in-laws. This is just a partial list of all the things many men fail to even acknowledge. With the keen perception of a detective, you can take notice and find a chance to say, "I *see* you. I see all that you're doing. Thank you." Then add her name at the end of that. Better yet, be like Q and help take some of the mental load off too.]

The Saintly Squadron versus The Brave Hearts Brigade

Don't let Rule No. 2 (Do things that show her you love her) confuse you about staying in the Saintly Squadron rather than moving to the Brave Hearts Brigade. Remember how I described the Saintly recruits as being ultra-diligent when it comes to helping out their partners? Mentally, they were operating from a "bartering" position, subconsciously thinking, "I will serve my partner and she will love and respect me in return." It was an unspoken *quid pro quo* in their heads. "I'll walk the dog, so that should make her excuse me for not helping with the dishes. I'll spend for a vacation, and that should cover my good deeds for the next few weeks."

That's not how it works for Jarvis, Q, and Alfred. The Brave Hearts do it to openly show they care about the relationship. They help above and beyond expectations because they know the success of the mission depends just as heavily on them as it does the main character. They aren't doing it to get a nod of thanks and a pat on the back. They do it because their role too is incredibly crucial and they know it. If they zone out or let the ball drop, the world ends.

That's what your partner would appreciate. Knowing that you've got her back in keeping the house together, looking after the kids, checking on everything else that could go wrong. Because she doesn't have a tribe of women helping her anymore. She has you.

Other Mental Brakes She Needs to Deal with on Her Own

Her mental brakes, by the way, aren't just the household chores. It could also be her silent resentments about something you did or forgot to do, or it could be as deep as her long-held attitude towards sex and its enjoyment. Was she raised to feel guilty about it? Has she explored her own body and learned what gives her pleasure? Is she self-conscious and uncomfortable being seen with her clothes off?

The previous chapter about knowing who you love is the avenue that will lead you to discovering these additional brakes. If she's been bottling up some ill feelings, she'll need to get them off her chest—and off her mind. To do this, you'll both need to learn how to express your feelings and discuss your boundaries calmly. Other things that make her feel uncomfortable or shy while having sex could be something you can find out once both of you become more open and vulnerable with each other. As for long-held attitudes regarding sex that may be constraining her, or if she's had bad experiences that she may not have told you or anyone else about, she may need counseling to help her process these incidents buried in her past.

Getting Things Going

The opposite of brakes would be her accelerants—those things that will help get her in the mood faster. Now that would be an interesting thing for the two of you to discover, because, as the writing in this area suggests, it's quite likely she hasn't given it that much thought on her own. That's to say, she may not have realized what she responds to sensually, besides the obvious, or explored her own body in an intimate way. Building that list together would be a fun thing to do. Does she like a certain cologne of yours? Is there music that turns her on? Would she enjoy a massage? Does she prefer the lights on or totally off? Are there certain words she would love to hear you whisper to get her in the mood? Would she like it if you were more aggressive? Gentler?

Put your Sherlock Holmes hat on and find her accelerants. Once you have a better idea about what slows her down and speeds her up, figure out how much time she needs for foreplay. A Glamour magazine survey of 1,000 women revealed that the majority engaged in nine minutes or less of foreplay, whereas a study[18] published in *The Journal of Sex Research* indicates that the ideal duration of foreplay for both men and women is significantly longer than the actual time being devoted to it.

Take note though, that I'm referring to what people traditionally refer to as foreplay—which is defined in the dictionary as the sexual activity that precedes intercourse. But after all that we've covered here about what gets a woman going, I believe you'll agree that there are three kinds of foreplay:

1. "In the moment" foreplay – this is foreplay as defined in the dictionary which, aside from the kissing and touching, should recruit her other accelerants right before you make love.

2. "In advance" foreplay – this is when you attend to the brakes in her head, way ahead of time; which means that you taking out the garbage on Wednesday, doing laundry on Thursday, and helping with dinner on Friday will lead to her being in the mood come Saturday.

3. "In her heart" foreplay – this is when you make her feel, every single day, that she's constantly on your mind, and that you value your relationship as much as your "other" full-time job (more on this in the next section).

I hope it's clear by now: Foreplay, in all its dimensions, begins right after your last orgasm and not ten minutes before you want your next one. To get to *third* base, you need all *three* kinds of foreplay.

And while we're on the subject of brakes and accelerants, let's talk a bit about lubrication. It's a common misconception that how wet a woman is signifies how ready she is for penetration. Even she might be surprised that this is not true. In much the same way that you can get an erection against your will, or that you can lose it or not even get one right when you really want one—a woman has no control over how wet she gets. She can be absolutely ready and still not be the least bit moist or be wet and slippery yet still not be in the mood. So for smooth operations, get yourself some water-based lubricant. Use the silicone-based variety if you fancy doing it in the shower or the tub.

This is particularly important if your partner has reached menopause; her body will not be as efficient in producing the natural lubrication needed. This is probably what has led to the misconception that women's interest in sex goes away after menopause. On the contrary, it crosses out one major thing from her mental list of concerns: the fear of getting pregnant. There is an eye-opening study conducted by Dan Buettner, an award-winning journalist, and his team on *blue zones,* a term that denotes places in the world where the world's oldest people live. The study reveals that in the blue zone region of Ikaria, Greece, about 80% of people between 65 and 100 years old are still having sex. Even more remarkable is that they're engaging in it without the help of sexual performance drugs. If your partner has been refusing sex because of the lack of lubrication leading to painful sex ever since menopause, then reach for that bottle of lubricant. But also, keep in mind, there's a huge chance it's not the menopause that's to blame for her lack of interest. It could be because there are not enough of all three kinds of foreplay.

She could be upset about your marriage, your neighborhood, her job; worried about finances, your daughter's grades, your son's tattoo; not happy with her body, your temper, your drinking; or any of a plethora of other concerns—pushing sex way, way down the list in her head of things that occupy her time.

Before we leave this topic, let me go back to the idea of your relationship being two people doing the tango. Even though you now understand how your partner is programmed to keep thinking of too many things all the time, and thus you'll be doing your best to adjust to that, she should also be doing her part in accepting the fact that you're programmed by your masculine biology to want and need sex far more than she does. It's part of your nature. Yes, you want more sex. And she should see how you want to have it with only one woman: Her. (Unless you have an agreement about having an open marriage—which, by the way, has a 92% failure rate.)

Hopefully, in accepting this about your physical makeup, she will stop resenting you and all other men because of the mantra she'd been fed ever since she hit puberty, when she was warned to "be careful of boys, because they only want one thing." Now that she's a grownup herself and is safely inside a relationship built on love and trust, she should understand and embrace your programming, and as one half of the tango, enjoy the dance with you.

Before we set off on our hike into the night, I pause to hand out something to add to our Knapsack of Knowledge. Having learned of the lessons I planned to impart on this leg of our journey, Q surprises us all with a gift. We each receive a Swiss Army knife with a diamond solitaire embedded in its handle. His card reads:

It's not the flashiness of your lifestyle that will put the sparkle in her eye. It's the hard work you put into your partnership that will make it last forever. — Q

(P.S. I had James Bond pay for the diamond.)

I hope you now have a better understanding as to why being her Q, Jarvis, or Alfred is going to help things in the bedroom—and every other place where it matters. What makes a man a hero in a woman's eyes is not the lavish vacations and precious gems and fancy dinner dates. It's all the little in-betweens that tell her you've got her back. When you anticipate her needs and make an effort to remember her likes and dislikes. Help her with the chores. Do things for her that a superhero would appreciate someone else doing. If she really is Wonder Woman, she'll do the same for you.

Be a Prince Charming that keeps on charming. Living happily ever after is hard work.

Rule No. 2: Do Things that Show Her You Love Her

Our journey takes us into the woods, and we immediately sight a handsome prince on a handsome white steed.

"Hark!" he calls out in his handsome voice. "Who goes there?"

"It's me," I say, "and a brigade of Brave Hearts on a quest to understand women."

"Ah, Brave Hearts indeed," he says, striking a royal pose on his gilded saddle. He does look charming, wearing a white velvet coat piped with golden cords, secured with ruby buttons. His britches and boots are ebony black, a red cape draped gracefully over his shoulders. "Alas, dear fellows. Your quest is far more challenging than mine. I'm off to slay a dragon!" He lofts his shiny sword towards the forest canopy.

"You're going to fight a dragon dressed like that?" I ask with a raise of my brows.

"Of course!" the prince replies. "That's what you call 'dating' in an enchanted forest. I'm going to slay a dragon so I can get the girl." A roar emanates from somewhere in the distance and his white stallion neighs, eager to gallop towards it. "I shall make sure I cross paths with you again," the prince declares before giving his horse free rein, "in the meantime, cheerio!"

The Mask of a Perfect Prince

To this day, children grow up with fairy tales that end right when the prince gets the girl. And the prince is always portrayed impeccably groomed and wearing his regal outfit, while the girl is either covered in cinders, playing housemaid to dwarves, beautifully sleeping her life away, or is stuck in a tower in dire need of a haircut. As the metaphor goes, a man ought to put on his royal charm when courting or wooing a girl so she would trust him enough and let him whisk her away from her sorry existence.

Unfortunately, when it comes to making first impressions, men still feel compelled to put on a mask as perfect as a prince, so the woman ends up falling for someone who's pretty close to a dream-come-true. Then after they're a couple, he relaxes his efforts of projecting near-perfection and waits for happily ever after to kick in.

That's how fairy tales with Prince Charming mislead young boys and girls with the illusion of an effortless happily-ever-after, as though going through the requisite displays of devotion before they become a couple is enough to keep the love going always and forever.

Here's how this translates into the real world.

Let's say a man notices a new co-worker, and she catches his interest. If he wants to get her interested in him, too, he'd have to step up his game.

If he always showed up at work in old tees and ill-fitting pants, he'd need to start wearing better-looking shirts and tighter jeans. He takes more time grooming himself in the morning and probably tosses a bottle of cologne in his gym bag and breath mints in the glove compartment, just in case. This is the period when she meets his Prince Charming version. The one who'll put on a blazer and take her out to fancy dinners and romantic dates, enchanting her by being extra attentive and thoughtful. Probably even sweet and ever-present. Texting her often and responding promptly enough.

If all things go well and his charm works, he "gets the girl." Both are blissful, and the relationship gets a label. In the story books, this is where the fairy tale says they live happily ever after. In the human world, this is when he reverts to normalcy. He settles back down to his plain old tees and skips the extra minute or two he'd been investing in front of the mirror in the morning. Before long, the attention he'd been giving her begins to dissipate. The texts and calls dwindle. His digital devices begin to invade their time alone—which have also become less frequent. After a while, the dates will probably be mostly her suggestion.

She notices the change, of course, which to the man's mind was only to be expected. Courtship was over. Time to head back to reality. But in her mind, though she knew he was out to impress her when he turned into Prince Charming, she also took it as a promise of things to come. That this prince was here for her and will someday be her king and she will be his queen.

Unfortunately, instead of keeping up the royal show, he relaxes instead and reveals himself to be a commoner. In the man's mind, he was putting on the charm just long enough to cast a spell, during which time she got to see the best he could be. Seriously, he wonders, how long do women expect us to keep up that perfect behavior?

The answer is: for as long as you want to live happily ever after. One of my clients summarized the reason for his divorce this way, "If you're going to put your best foot forward, you'd better be sure you can keep that damn foot in front of you for the rest of your life."

[Women, of course, have to do their share of not pretending to be someone they're not. During the courtship period, they can be perfectly radiant, perpetually agreeable, and blind to all your flaws until they turn into your mother, principal, or boss. That's when they could turn an accusing finger at you and say the change in their attitude was mainly triggered by the shift in your behavior. But all this is a subject for another book—one addressed to women. For this one, let's focus on this side of the fence.]

Now, here's probably the only dating tip you'll find in this book: Become the prince she would want to be with for the rest of her life. Introduce her to the best version of yourself that you can realistically sustain—and once you start courting her, do things that you can keep doing indefinitely. Stay charming and keep courting her—as long as you both shall live.

I can't count how many men in the throes of newfound love have declared, "She makes me want to be a better man." And they embrace the hard work of living up to that standard. So my question is: If it takes a better man to get the woman who he wants to spend the rest of his life with, should he stop being that better man he made himself into when the "rest of their lives" begin?

This is nuts, you probably think. The reason why it's called "courtship" is because there's a time frame. It is a period of wooing. In the animal kingdom, courtship is defined as "behavior that occurs before and during mating, often including elaborate displays." Peacocks fan out their tails just long enough to catch the eye of a mate. That's how nature does it! It, therefore, cannot be logically sustained because human males need to get back to work, back to their friends, get on with their lives, and not keep up with lifelong elaborate displays. Most of all, they have a mission.

Which is precisely why I prescribe not doing anything during courtship which you cannot sustain indefinitely. Because unlike most lower animals who impregnate and run, you, highly evolved human sir, are expected to stick around for a very long time, ideally monogamously, because of a commitment inspired by love.

Things have changed. Kro-ah, in the caveman era, was only looking for a man who, because of his physique and repute as a hunter or warrior, seemed to have good seed and was strong enough to protect and provide for her and their brood. In contrast, Kro-ah's female descendants (the productive, emotionally mature ones) have complete and fulfilling lives and are open to sharing that life with men who will make it feel sweeter.

In fairy tales, the prince finds a seemingly ordinary girl who later turns into a Disney Princess. In real life—in real evolutionary life, her DNA hasn't really changed. She is still, for the most part, Kro-ah. Still willing to do the hard work for home and hearth, be a loving mother to her children and the devoted wife and lover to her man. And yet, the prince is finding it harder and harder to find ordinary girls trapped in towers, cleaning up cinders, or beautifully sleeping their lives away.

So what changed? Her brain didn't get bigger; she was just given access to better education. Her ego didn't get bloated, she was simply encouraged to dream and have ambitions. And because of these two changes, she gained the confidence and capacity to make a living and fend for herself. That doesn't mean her heart grew cold. On the contrary, she got to realize she deserved a warmer man.

The Fairy Tale Magic of Romance

In my advertising class exercise, where I had male students come up with the Unique Selling Proposition (USP) for women so that men would want them imported onto an all-male planet, I'd also asked the young women to come up with the USP for men so that women would be interested in having them share their all-heterosexual-female planet for the purpose of marriage, as you'll remember being mentioned earlier. As with the men, sex and procreation were not included, given that babies were delivered by storks. Interestingly, their initial answers were related to brawn. That is, they would want the men around for security and protection. But then I'd point out that their planet had an all-female army and cops and fire brigades etc. So I asked them if they just wanted the men around so they could get married to personal bodyguards. And then they'd give answers like companionship, adventure, fun times—things that I'd point out they were currently having with their female friends on their planet.

As I had done with their male classmates, I reminded them of the main criterion of the exercise. The USP needed to be *unique* in that it was something another heterosexual female cannot give them. Once focused on that requirement, one way or another, the groups all came up with variations on the same answer: Romance.

It's what makes an ordinary bouquet of flowers mean something more. It makes dining out special. A necklace, a box of chocolates, a handwritten letter—all become more than just jewelry, candy, and a note. They become symbols of love. Even taking out the trash and helping with the dishes become acts of love when *you* do them. (Imagine what it means when you don't.)

To put it simply: You can't spell ROMANCE without a MAN.

When the all-female groups presented their conclusions to the class, invariably the young men would scoff at the answer. Saying something in the lines of, "Is that how shallow you are?"

To silence the verbal combat that usually ensues between the boys and girls after that, I mentioned the statistic that 80% of divorces were asked for by women. Then I asked, "Do you suppose it might have something to do with men thinking that romance is shallow?"

The young men would then shake their heads, saying it was something too hard to keep up for life. I just tell them to remember this class exercise, and that hopefully it would be a lesson they'd remember when they're married, and their wife didn't seem so happy anymore.

In case you're thinking, "Yeah, sure. Romance. What else would you expect from a bunch of co-eds?" I have also had conversations with women in their thirties and from every decade thereafter up to their eighties who echo the same sentiment. One of them said, "Your next book, make the title, "Men, please watch chick flicks."" Another one said, "I want what's in the movies." And these are successful women who are either in high-flying corporate jobs or retired from top management posts. Romance is not a childhood fantasy for little women. It's something smart, mature women have seen many women receive from their loving men—and not just in the movies. They themselves received it when the men they fell in love with were still trying to win their hearts.

If, after being drawn to a confident, successful, independent woman, a man pulls away in doubt, asking himself, "How do I fit into her world?" then he should imagine her world without him. Without the magic of romance in her life, she becomes ... a lot like everyone else who's single and unattached. Feeling that life is good—and yet, maybe, things could be better ... if they found someone who felt like home.

Let me be clear that romance is not about mimicking the superficial courtship rituals of candlelit dinner dates and showing up with flowers. If that's all you imagine it to be, then that indeed would be shallow. Allow me to share with you the fundamentals of how to speak the language of Romance in ways she will finally appreciate. (Yes, the word Romance is capitalized for a reason, which I'll explain in the next section.)

The Language of Romance

If I were to come up with an "alphabet" that will form your expressions of love, it will be through *Thoughtfulness*. It is the bedrock on which the language of Romance stands.

Thoughtfulness is defined as the characteristic or habit of anticipating and being attentive to the needs and interests of others. Let's emphasize that and restate it within our context: *The language of Romance, which is Thoughtfulness, is the habit of anticipating and being attentive to her needs and interests.*

Showing up with red roses may be considered romantic, but giving her pink carnations instead because that's her favorite flower in her favorite color makes it Romantic with a capital R because you have given it *thought*. This means, Romance that is thoughtful is specific to your partner, making your choices intentional. It's about knowing her favorites, dream destinations and staycations, most wanted lists, and personal preferences. Dark or white chocolate? Red or white wine? Marvel or DC? Paperbacks or eBooks?

An important note is that this rule, which is Rule No. 2 (Do things that show her you love her) is hinged on you having done your part with Rule No. 1 (Know who you love and why). If you've accomplished your assignment as Sherlock Holmes and have had deep conversations with her, you now know her likes and dislikes, understand her desires and goals, and can anticipate what she needs and what would interest her—then you're equipped to proceed.

A Thoughtful Action Plan

On the assumption that a man is typically not so in touch with his emotions, is action oriented, and thinks more than he feels, I've put together a manual that harnesses those thoughts and translates them into an action plan that will crystallize his feelings. One could say it's like a step-by-step guide on how to speak the Romantic language of Thoughtfulness introduced above.

The following "action plan" is organized under three key roles you play in her life—that of Friend, Lover, and Partner—that serve as counterparts to the same roles that are important for her to play in your life. Once again, it corresponds to the trine of the heart, body, and mind.

- FRIEND – Because friendship is what makes the heart grow fonder, and strong relationships are what bring us happiness.

- LOVER – Because our bodies need a daily dose of hugs, kisses, and warm embraces for our overall well-being and for our emotional intimacy to grow stronger.

- PARTNER – Because when our minds think as one when we support each other's goals and make decisions around shared values, life itself feels a lot lighter.

The Role of Friend

Perhaps the best marital advice I've heard as regards choosing a life partner is to marry your best friend. It's quite a disadvantage that most romantic relationships begin driven by hormones and lust. It makes it quite a challenge to transition that into friendship. Lust clouds your judgment and tempts you to ignore and forgive hurtful or inconsiderate behavior because you don't want to lose the high of mutual attraction.

Maybe that's why arranged marriages have a better batting average at success than love marriages. According to the 2023 Gitnux Marketdata Report, around 55% of marriages in the world are arranged, meaning their partners were chosen by their families. (Note that this is different from a forced marriage, though sometimes the two are indistinguishable. Arranged marriages have the consent of the couple. Forced marriage is not my topic here.)

The global divorce rate for arranged marriages is 4% to 6%. In India, where about 90% of marriages are arranged, the divorce rate is only 1%. Compare those to the divorce rate in the United States of around 40% to 50%. One could say that culture, religion, and legal restrictions play a huge part in these statistics. But a study by psychologists Usha Gupta and Pushpa Singh of the University of Rajasthan used Rubin's Love and Liking Scale and put that notion to the test. The scale, as the name suggests, assesses the intensity of liking and loving in a romantic relationship, and its results reveal love in love marriages tends to start high and declines rather quickly. In contrast, love in the arranged marriages examined by the researchers started out low and gradually increased. After five years, they surpassed the level in love marriages. A decade into the arranged marriage, the love was nearly twice as strong.

The assumption is that, in an arranged marriage, the partners barely know a thing about each other, so they take their time to understand their spouse, observing things, learning, and making adjustments to make the marriage work. In addition, these marriages are generally arranged by loved ones who know the individuals well—their values, upbringing, and personalities—so the matches could well be guided by an objective assessment of how the two might jibe even before they meet (as opposed to relationships sparked by physical attraction).

I know I said the best advice was "Marry your best friend," which is the farthest thing a partner in an arranged marriage is. But the couples there go into the union with minimal expectations, and they accept the other person as they are. They walk into the union prepared to give the relationship hard work, and they begin by becoming good friends. This eliminates our fairytale problem of a Prince Charming and Princess Darling who started out dating as better versions of themselves, resulting in complaints later on that the awesome person they met is different from the person they married.

With love marriages, despite knowing that real life is no fairy tale, couples still can't help but count on ... well, love when things get rocky. But love without friendship is even rockier ground; it might even lead to more hard knocks than solid ground. Which is why I've given the example of arranged marriages as a means of encouraging you to make a great friend of your partner if you aren't best friends yet. And here are some thoughtful things to do to solidify that friendship.

A. Words: In the bestselling book *The 5 Love Languages: The Secret to Love That Lasts*, author Gary Chapman has words of affirmation as one of those languages. The others are gifts, physical touch, acts of service, and quality time. Most people may have come to associate these languages solely with romantic love, but they are highly applicable to friendships as well. With the goal of making our life partner our best friend, we should see that expressing our love in these various forms begins at the grass roots of our relationship.

To strengthen our bond, Chapman advises that we uncover our partner's love language and then "speak" to them in that language. In the context of a romantic relationship, not deciphering what's being said can lead to unmet emotional needs. Let's say your wife expresses her love through acts of service by keeping the house clean, whereas you couldn't care less if the house grew messy in a month for as long as you had sex twice a week because your love language is through touch. Or maybe you keep showering her with new clothes and jewelry because gifts are how you express your affection, but what she would value more is quality time, like you hiring a babysitter so the two of you can have a night together without the kids.

It's good advice to know how your partner expresses their love best and how they wish to receive yours in the most appropriate way to them. Which is why all five of those love languages are somehow reflected and subsumed within the nine thoughtful expressions of Romance prescribed in this book. It's particularly helpful if you've been missing the target all this time because you've been completely omitting the language with which your partner understands love. For instance, what if she would like to receive love literally through words that affirm her value to you, and yet you seldom, if ever, say what you feel whenever she smiles at you and makes your heart flutter, when she does something special—or even when she performs mundane tasks that help make your day-to-day easier.

A major difference between Chapman's advice and mine is that I prescribe that you use *all* the expressions of Thoughtfulness that make up the language of Romance—daily, as much as possible (except gift-giving, perhaps, although frequency and meaning—rather than monetary value—is encouraged). Even if your partner says they appreciate being shown love a specific way, focusing on just that alone could create an area of concentrated warmth but leave a lot of cold spots elsewhere in your relationship. Because, for instance, your language of love is physical touch, and when your partner learns this, she becomes more receptive to your advances and also initiates more often, but then she doesn't give you words of affirmation that let you know how much she appreciates what you do and never gives you words of praise even after you've gone the extra mile to impress her. Wouldn't that leave you wanting? Or what if it's the reverse; that she constantly praises and lauds you on social media, but once you're alone together, she's always too tired or has a headache or minds the household chores more than you. Or maybe you learn that she wants more quality time together, and you grant her that by taking her out one special evening, but you don't say a word all night about how pretty she looks or how much you appreciate having her in your life. That gap somehow diminishes the quality of that time, even if you spend it with no one else but her. That's why I advise that all these expressions of Thoughtfulness be spread throughout your days and nights. The different roles you play as friend, lover, and partner will be like the triple helix of the DNA of your union. And perhaps the most obvious and expected way of expressing one's feelings is literally with words.

Research has shown that even between friends, an unexpected call or text is valued far more by the recipient than what is predicted by the sender. So the simple act of sending a surprise text that expresses a positive thought or feeling (not about something you forgot or asking a favor or a question about a chore) in the middle of a workday will work its own little touch of magic that can brighten your partner's hectic afternoon. Friends do that for each other. So do workmates. Between romantic partners, such words become much more meaningful.

It seems simple enough for any man to know the value of hearing the words, "I love you." Earlier, I'd mentioned a study that suggested how saying it with the person's name ("I love you, Chris" versus just "I love you") deepened the effect of the statement. Yet oftentimes, we omit the name, and even drop the I. And sometimes, even the you. So oftentimes we just toss out, "Love ya," then rush out the door.

Thoughtful Words are about saying things genuinely—and frequently—from the heart. When you express your love, gratitude, appreciation, admiration, support, and encouragement with words, you crystallize your sentiments that could be missed or taken for granted. This is probably an aspect in your relationship you've somewhat overlooked, because for men, actions speak louder than words. But for women, you could have spent the day working from home so you could do some laundry, order pizza for lunch, walk the dog, cook dinner, then clean up the kitchen because she's been feeling sick since morning. Then when evening comes, she might end up telling you how upset she was because you hadn't said a word all day that expressed how concerned you were about how she was feeling. In your language, you were saying "I love you. I hope you feel better" all day long. But all she understood was that you spent your day at home because you had so many things to attend to.

So make your intentions crystal clear. Say all the good things you're feeling and thinking. Compliment her if you like how she looks in her outfit, or if the pie she made was delicious even though she'd made it many times before. Say you appreciate having her come over and hug you in silence at the end of a long hard day. Or look in her eyes and tell her that you still find her gorgeous after all these years. She might be blind to the meaning behind everything you're doing. Or she may want to know the reasons why you still love her. So say it. Just say it. Often.

B. Gifts: It's normal for friends to give each other presents, even when there's no occasion. Like a T-shirt with a silly print on it. A cup from Starbucks. Some donuts when they pop by. All these are Thoughtful Gifts given to a friend who they know would laugh at that stupid shirt and would appreciate the coffee and sweets because it's exactly the kind they like. And these gifts are given with no other agenda than to see a smile light up their face. I don't think there's any man who hasn't, at one time or another, given his partner a gift as a symbol of his affection. What makes a *Thoughtful Gift* different from all other kinds of gifts? The fact that it is given with careful consideration of her personal desires—with no ulterior motive besides wanting to give her joy. By ulterior motive here, I mean it's not used to buy his way out of having to give her more of himself.

Even if you splurge on a lavish vacation—she's not going to be "bribed" into believing that's what you call "attention" if you don't pay her any mind most of the time. A pearl necklace doesn't replace a string of words that express your love, admiration, and appreciation. Giving her free rein on a shopping spree doesn't take the place of spending quality time with her, neither does it buy you freedom to neglect and ignore her or not help her around the house. Nor should that lavish spa day simply be a ticket to get what you want in bed.

Gifts *without* thoughtfulness are calorie-loaded cakes and ice cream you bring home even though she's on a diet. It's buying her that purple shirt you thought looked cute on the mannequin, even though there's not a single purple thing in her closet. It's surprising her with a party with a huge banner saying "Happy 40th Birthday" even though she doesn't want anyone knowing her real age.

A friend of mine recently told me how her husband had bought most of her new paperbacks, even after she expressed no desire for them. "He'd give me logical reasons why I ought to like the books, and then he'd buy them anyway." It's easy to assume he was buying the gifts out of love, but he wasn't being thoughtful—the right way.

What's important is that you listen, observe, and most of all, remember. It's that shoulder bag you got her because you went out shopping with her once, and she mentioned how much she liked it but thought it was too pricey—so you bought it without her knowing. It's those potted mums you brought home for her because she loves to garden and prefers living plants over cut flowers. It's buying her sugar-free cakes and ice cream because you want to help her stay on her diet.

Thoughtful Gifts are given even when there's nothing to celebrate and no special occasion. They're gifts, and they're thoughtful. They're tailor-made simply to please her.

C. Freedom: The playwright Anton Chekhov wrote, "If you are afraid of loneliness, don't marry." Rather than assume he personally made a wrong choice in life, I'd like to think that he believed married couples tend to wall themselves up away from friends and relatives, concentrating on their insular lives as a couple and their family unit. These same friends and relatives also instinctively invite married people less to get-togethers, believing they've already got calendars full of couple-type activities.

The thing about friendships is that no matter how close you get, there remains a sense of belonging without feeling that you are "owned" or are dependent. As friends, both of you are fully aware of this other person who deserves a special place in our lives, yet shares you with many others. And this freedom is something inherent to friendships—that you see yourself as separate from the other, free to have your own set of beliefs, a different calendar, and even sets of friends different from theirs. Such a dynamic allows the friendship to enrich your life rather than constrain it.

The *Thoughtful Freedom* of friendship helps both of you to meet your psychological need for novelty and variety as individuals, and the benefits will spill over into your intimate lives as well. Science provides evidence that couples with greater self-expansion—that is, pursuing self-growth through new and exciting life experiences—have better relationships. A 2020 study highlights how women with low desire who increased their level of self-expansion reported higher desire, greater sexual satisfaction, and felt more affectionate and satisfied with their relationship.[19]

As your friendship grows more and more stable and comfortable, stave off relationship boredom. Having the freedom to pursue individual and independent interests will help keep things interesting.

When you did the exercise of going through your self-growth pillars to get to know yourself better, we reviewed the state of your social life. The reason we did that is because, based on the Harvard study on happiness, the quality of one's relationships—all kinds, not just the romantic ones—contribute the most to a person's happiness. So encourage your partner to enjoy her freedom with her friends and family. Or, if she'd rather indulge in some alone time to relish life on her own, give her that freedom too.

Is it possible to grant her freedom that isn't thoughtful? Yes, if you send out vibes of suspicion or jealousy despite you letting her go out without you. Or you only urge her to get time away as a means of bargaining for more freedom for yourself. (What if she doesn't want to spend any time away from you? Go back to finding out why that is. She might be subconsciously seeing you as the answer to a hidden issue, like a core wound she needs to heal. Too much time together can be a red flag towards co-dependency.)

The Role of Lover

When it comes to the stark differences between the sexes, here's one more thing our science and biology teachers didn't put much emphasis on: How our reproductive instincts could affect our romantic partnerships.

Once you hit puberty, you start producing several million sperm per day. Although the entire cycle of spermatogenesis takes approximately two and a half months, about 1,500 sperm are born every second. Once inside the female reproductive tract, sperm can survive for five days and it only takes one to produce a child. So technically speaking, provided you have healthy sperm, you're capable of getting a woman pregnant every time you ejaculate.

Compare this with women who are born with their entire life's supply of ova. After puberty, her ovaries will release a mature ovum, typically, once a month. It travels down her fallopian tube and stays there for half a day to a day and a half. Strictly speaking, it's an average of only one day a month where there's an egg just hanging around, waiting to be fertilized. But combining that with the five-day lifespan of the sperm inside a woman's body, there's a six-day "fertile window" when intercourse can result in pregnancy. Technically speaking, she can have sex all she wants every day, but she's only capable of getting pregnant once within that fertile window per month (excluding the rare occasions her ovaries don't follow the schedule). Pregnancy can happen even if she doesn't climax.

Even if she's not aroused. Even if the sex is against her will. But only within that window.

If she does conceive, her uterus becomes fully occupied for nine months thereafter. And given the mind- and body-altering aftereffects of having a human being leave her body through her vagina, plus her postpartum hormones, breastfeeding, and round-the-clock duties as a mother, she's not likely to be eager to hop into bed with you again for quite a while.

Considering how nature designed things, is it any wonder then why men are biologically driven to want far more sex than women do? Nature finds no benefit in driving a woman to expend energy on an act that won't result in procreation. She experiences increased libido approaching ovulation as the amount of the hormone estrogen rises to its peak—then drops after ovulation occurs.

You might say the invention of the pill should have changed how the female body responds to her hormones and how her mind regards unplanned pregnancies. But the likelihood of pregnancy isn't the only factor to be considered here. There's also the *un*likelihood of an orgasm. Even there, you have a far greater batting average. Heterosexual men report to have orgasms 95% of the time during partnered sexual activity, but for women, the figure ranges from only 50 to 70%, depending on the study. In a survey published in 2018[20] involving women ages 18 to 94, only about 18% reported achieving orgasm from intercourse alone. There are also studies revealing that 5 to 15% of women have yet to experience an orgasm, while 59% admitted to faking one at one time or another.[21]

So now do you better understand why I advise three kinds of foreplay? It's not about her not loving you enough or being too moody or hormonal. Billy Crystal, playing the character Mitch Robbins in the movie *City Slickers* said, "Women need a reason to have sex, men just need a place." He was right. Women need a reason to have sex. So if you're not a Thoughtful Lover, what's in it for her?

Sex is usually not a comfortable topic to discuss. But if you've become the best of friends, it shouldn't be that difficult to steer the conversation in that direction. It's very important that Rule No. 1 is applied here—that of knowing the woman you love when it comes to her desires and dislikes when making love. There is no one-size-fits-all manual for In-the-Moment foreplay and what women want sexually. One woman may want it slow with soft and gentle kisses; another may prefer it rough and raw. One could be turned on by dirty talk, another could be driven to ecstasy by your tender words of love and compliments about her beauty. Your key to great sex, therefore, is open communication.

On a more general scope, here are a few things you can keep in mind to become a better lover.

A. Presentation: In the culinary world, there's no question how important presentation is in making a dish mouthwatering. And if you want your woman drooling at the sight of you, then you'd better give your presentation serious consideration.

Men know what it takes to look good for a business presentation. There's a standard he aims for to be seen as respectable and impressive. In comparison, how much thought do you give to how you dress to impress her? Are you just aiming for presentable?

I'd like to call attention to the huge gap between an impressive presentation of yourself and being merely presentable. Presentable simply means "to be socially acceptable, passable, or sufficiently good." That sounds almost just a notch above being barefoot in pajamas.

Honestly, if you were to ask someone to describe a potential blind date, I doubt you'd be all that interested in meeting her if the best they could muster is, "She's presentable."

Surely, there must be something in between being dressed for the big guns and being just presentable for your partner. Unfortunately, presentable is how high the bar goes for a lot of men when it comes to dressing up. Numerous studies have demonstrated that women are drawn to men that are well dressed. And by well-dressed, I mean showing up dressed appropriately for the occasion.

Simply put, dressing sharp makes you the opposite of dull. Taking charge of how you look shows people you can call the shots. Consider who you will be seeing and interacting with and how you want them to respond to you. What you wear and how you choose to present yourself reflects how you want to be treated, and it will influence whether others listen to you, trust, and respect you. Whether it's a formal dinner, a business conference, or your kid's basketball game, there's a way of presenting yourself that lets you cut a fine figure. Even when just lazing at home, looking sloppy and smelling like yesterday won't help impress the lady of the house. (Believe it or not, I've had clients, male and female, complaining about how their partners simply stopped bothering to look good for them, citing this as one major reason for them ending the union.)

Results of the Well-Dressed Men Survey conducted by Kelton Research reveal that well-dressed men are viewed as sexier, more well-liked, smarter, more successful—and also fare better in relationships. More than that, 91% of respondents in the US survey think dressing well can make a man appear to be more physically attractive than he really is. And yet, so few men are well-dressed these days. Let's say he and his girlfriend are going out on a date, she could be wearing a very flattering dress, makeup with a nice hairstyle, and really nice shoes. And the man she's with? He could be in shorts, a sports shirt, rubber shoes, and a baseball cap. That makes him presentable. And in her eyes, maybe not exactly sexy, confident, attractive, or classy (reported as the top traits women perceive in a well-dressed man). I'm not saying you always have to dress to the nines, but if you want her to expend the effort to always look good for you, then the least you can do is return the favor.

During one exercise in my advertising class when we were dealing with a fashion brand, I asked my male students if they would like to dress better than they currently did when going out. Most of them did, and some even admitted to regularly browsing the internet to look at photos of how to be a well-dressed man. They liked what they saw, and could afford it, too, but they still just went with what others usually wore around town. If you drill down to the fundamental reason? It wasn't a lack of money, time, or ideas. It was a lack of confidence, their sense of self-worth, and a need to "belong" with everyone else.

This takes us back to the exercise we had about self-love. There is a pillar of self-growth which is about your physical state—covering your health, hygiene, looks and so on. If you assessed yourself as "Really Good" there, I hope this included your presentation. And what does *Thoughtful Presentation* entail? It involves knowing what she considers more appealing on you. Does she prefer seeing you with a week-long stubble instead of clean-shaven? Without dry, chapped lips? With that particular scent of deodorant and her favorite cologne. Boxers or briefs? Jeans or shorts? Loose shirts or tight ones? As her lover, think of yourself as a well-dressed gift she can hardly wait to unwrap.

When you walk into a room, you want to feel proud of the woman you're with. Believe me, she wants to feel the same about you. (If, on the other hand, it's your lady who isn't expending any effort on her physique and presentation, then take advantage of every chance you get to compliment her on her appearance. If such a chance hardly ever arises, then I suggest you find an opportune and appropriate time to bring up how it makes you feel when she seems oblivious to how she grooms herself or dresses up for you. There's more on how to do this in the section about the Incredible Hulk and how to manage conflict without anger entering the picture.)

Take care of your physique. Practice good hygiene. Dress well. Smell good. Even when it's just the two of you. Or rather, especially when it's just the two of you. The irony you'll experience as her lover is that being well-dressed will make her want to tear your clothes off.

B. Togetherness: Comedian Patrice O'Neal once quipped, "Men want to be alone … but not by ourselves." That encapsulates the sentiment quite clearly of how a man wants to be in a relationship but with enough free space left around him so he doesn't feel stifled, controlled, or engulfed. This, however, leaves the woman wondering, "How do I show you I care if we're not together? And how can you say you love me if you don't like being with me? Do you even think of me when we're apart?"

When it comes to spending quality time with a romantic partner, a study published in the European Review of Applied Psychology[22] found that women favor communication, affection, and emotional closeness more compared to men who are more inclined to share activities or have joint leisure time with their partner. Adding to this mismatch in inclinations is the finding of the US National Survey of Families and Households that the less time couples spend together, the less sex they have. Both are pretty good reasons why you need to put a lot more thought into your togetherness.

Thoughtful Togetherness is about spending time with each other in meaningful ways. "Plain" togetherness is, like, taking the dog for a walk with your partner but you hardly exchange any words. Or the two of you sitting next to each other while watching TV but are minding your phones' notifications more than each other. "Forced" togetherness is when you get dragged to a family gathering of hers where you feel like an outsider, or when she grudgingly goes with you to the gym for a workout she doesn't really want to do. Togetherness "Overload" is when you end up sacrificing time with family and friends, personal hobbies, and time alone, bordering on or even entering into co-dependency. There's a sweet spot to time spent together that allows both of you to grow as individuals and as a couple. You'll need to determine that sweet spot for yourselves.

What's valuable is spending enough time together in meaningful ways that deepen and strengthen your relationship. Research has shown that it's not the amount of time but the quality of that time that matters; individuals who reported spending more time interacting with their partner also reported greater experienced closeness.[23] (Keep in mind, though, that for couples experiencing high levels of distress, spending more time together may not be helpful because it might only lead to more conflict. For such couples, learning how to communicate better first would be ideal.)

Given everything else that's going on in our lives, scheduling a date once a week is highly advised, and that means gadgets aside and no talk about work, the kids, and household concerns. If circumstances make physical time together impossible, then have a pleasant talk online—not about chores and work and the news but about the person in front of you who is your best friend.

A study from the National Bureau of Economic Research reveals that people who consider their spouse to be their best friend are nearly compared to those who don't. The Thoughtful-Togetherness kind of date puts importance on what happens between the two of you—stripped of the scenery, activity, or occasion.

Ask her questions! From those seemingly frivolous ones you'd ask on a first date to deeper ones that will help you navigate the future. Here are a few to get you started:

- If you could have any superpower, what would it be and why?
- What did love look like between your parents when you were a child?
- What would you change about yourself if you could?
- What's your favorite date that we've ever been on?
- Have you learned anything new about yourself since we got together?
- What's something you're really proud of?
- Are there any topics you're still nervous about bringing up with me?
- What are your beliefs about the afterlife?
- What do I do that's guaranteed to make you smile?

Try something new together. Stay overnight at a new place. Go on an adventure. Try to go to bed at the same time regularly. Cuddle after making love. (A new study says cuddling after sex makes the experience significantly better for her.)

If all you can really afford to do in terms of time is just walk the dog together, then make it count. Make your time together matter. Ask meaningful questions and deepen your understanding of how she and you are different from who you were just the other day.

C. Contact: This can mean eye contact, hugging, kissing, sex, or simply touching and holding hands. What makes these things *Thoughtful Contact* is that they are intentional and are more than just "going through the motions?" When you look into each other's eyes, sex turns into making love. Hugging for at least 20 seconds makes the physical contact long enough for the body to release oxytocin—a hormone that triggers feelings of love and closeness. Instead of a quick peck on the cheek when you leave for work, make it a six-second kiss on the lips. According to relationship coach Dr. John Gottman, lengthening kisses to six seconds creates a moment of connection with our partner; it pauses your brain long enough for you to focus on your partner and could be key to having a better relationship.

What makes Togetherness different from Contact? Togetherness is time spent in a way that deepens emotional intimacy. You can be together physically but not make much physical contact. Inversely, a couple can engage in a lot of sexual activity and not forge deep emotional bonds. Contact creates the physical connection that turns emotional intimacy sparked during time together into electricity arcing between lovers.

Contact After the Kids Come Along

Getting enough Thoughtful Contact in the early stages of a relationship is practically effortless, but it tends to diminish after the so-called honeymoon phase and turns into a challenge after the kids come along.

This can become a problem, particularly for the man in a relationship, who could end up with touch starvation, also called affection deprivation or skin hunger. This can happen when he doesn't get enough physical contact, which can make him stressed, anxious, and/or depressed.

Our need for contact begins at birth. Within hours, newborns gaze at their mothers' faces, and in a couple of months, babies begin to direct their eyes more intentionally and stare at their caregivers as a means to communicate. A new study finds that when a baby makes eye contact with an adult, their brainwaves fall in sync, paving the way for better communication. Doctors also suggest that the mother hold and carry her baby often to promote the child's healthy development. We all need a constant dose of positive physical contact, and this need for human touch goes on throughout our lives.

At the beginning of every romantic relationship, a couple gets this need fulfilled—and then some. But when the baby comes, there's something the couple doesn't realize. Mom spends her day constantly carrying, kissing, breastfeeding, hugging, cuddling her newborn, and thus gets her much-needed daily dose of skin and eye-to-eye contact from her baby. When her husband comes home, he's still hungry for some touch but she's fully sated. And exhausted. Leading to the superficial types of contact between husband and wife thereafter. Add to this how the woman prioritizes her role as mother from then on and puts the roles of lover and girlfriend on the back burner. She still plays the role of wife—who looks after her husband and their home—but the tonality of that role is far from the Romantic connection we're hoping to keep alive.

Adequate doses of physical contact are essential yet rare for an unpartnered man to get; it's highly unlikely that the few handshakes at work, the thumps on the back, and quick bro hugs from his buddies are enough to fill his body's needs. What can the man do to compensate when his touch-sated wife is in no mood for kisses and cuddles? He spends his free time playing with and hugging the kids, or even the pets, while he lets her get some rest. Hopefully, he doesn't go outside the home and outside the marriage to get his health-giving dose of human touch.

Thoughtful Contact makes touching, kissing, hugging, and looking into each other's eyes a deliberate and mindful act, several times a day.

Every day. Have a talk with your partner about this and help her see how the world of touch is far more open for women than it is for men.

The Role of Partner

Oftentimes, when partnership in marriage is discussed, it leads to discussions of equality and dividing expenses, responsibilities, and chores 50:50. But that's not how real partnerships work. Even among business partnerships, assignments aren't divided equally down the middle. The division of responsibilities is assessed, discussed, and agreed upon, and that's the same process a couple should go through when their two lives merge. Partnership is a division of "assignments" that both parties are amenable, comfortable, and happy with.

Unfortunately, it's a step many couples skip. Maybe out of awkwardness, shyness, or sheer oversight. In my case, it was mainly ignorance that caused us to walk into marriage in our twenties without a proper discussion about how we planned to manage bank accounts, household responsibilities, bills, childcare and so on. And given how we both avoided conflict and difficult conversations during our marriage, it's no wonder the marital house fell asunder.

Beyond agreements made beforehand, partnership also entails initiative and consideration. Not everything can be foreseen. Not everything will fall into place as planned. So adjustments will need to be made. And a lot of times, it will be greatly appreciated when the changes are volunteered out of understanding and compassion. Those are the times when you truly feel your partner has your back.

What follows are the thoughtful ways your role as partner can become part of the language of Romance.

A. Attention: Great partnerships work when you're mindful of the other person's needs. Can you imagine what would happen if Robin was oblivious to Batman. If Watson didn't mind Sherlock? If Maverick ignored Goose? (I know, Goose died, but it's not because Maverick wasn't paying him any attention.)

Thoughtful Attention means taking notice of someone in a way that matters to them. Say it's your wife's "duty" to fold the laundry, but she sighs and mentions that she needs to finish a Keynote presentation for tomorrow, so you step up and say you'll take care of the laundry. Or maybe she always takes care of the grocery expenses, but after she mutters something about how much supermarket prices have gone up, you remember she's been wanting to get herself a new laptop for quite a while. So you tell her you can take over the groceries for the time being.

Surprisingly, one "need" that constantly needs attention is the need for attention itself! Such as when you show up feeling exhausted and your partner asks what you'd like to do to recharge. Or if you come home still energized from work and she asks, "What's up?" then eagerly listens to you talk about your win that day. Imagine those situations reversed, and that's you giving her the attention she needs. Being part of a team means you always feel noticed and seen—because you can sense that your presence, how you feel, and what you say matters.

Thoughtful Attention, therefore, could be as simple as responding nicely when your partner points out a puppy trotting by.

"Oh, look! How cute!" she might exclaim.

And you'd turn and look towards the little dog and say, "Yeah, what breed is that?" As opposed to you glancing and not saying a thing or grunting and not even looking.

This situation is an example of what the psychologist John Gottman calls a "bid for attention" which he considers a fundamental unit of emotional connection. When your partner sends out a bid, it signifies a desire to connect. Respond to it, and you tighten your bonds. Turn away and it's a relationship killer.

Some bids are crystal clear, like outright calls for help or a whispered request for something special you'd like in the bedroom. Some are a bit hazy, like a fleeting pout or a heavy sigh. Thoughtful Attention is about being attentive and responsive to these bids.

Is it possible to give unthinking or thoughtless attention? Yes, when the response one gives shows her he forgot something important about her. Say, when she pointed out the cute puppy walking by, the man asks, "You want me to get you one?" Forgetting that she's allergic to dogs despite liking them. There's also such a thing as unwanted attention, of course. It's one that goes against their grain. You may be the recipient of this when your woman dotes on you like a mother. Or comments on your behavior or outfit negatively as a way to show she cares.

Pay attention to her bids and respond in a way that matters to her. Research has shown that high responsiveness is one of the best predictors of long-term happiness in romantic relationships.[24] Compared to those who get divorced, couples who stay happily married are often more responsive to their partner's needs.

B. Deeds: What everyone looks for in a partner is someone you can rely on to act for the benefit of the team. And because Rule No. 2 is about doing things that show her you love her, this entire chapter explains how this translates to an expression of Romance.

Thoughtful Deeds are acts of love that encompass both what's expected of you and the things you do beyond that. This echoes Gary Chapman's acts of service as one of the five love languages. One difference here though is how I suggest we call them. I've had a few people react to the phrase "Acts of Service" as having an undertone of subservience, almost like what a butler does for the owners of the house. Thoughtful Deeds, in comparison, reflects the mindful nature of the language of Romance you wish to maintain in a healthy relationship.

If it's really your assignment to cook dinner every night, it becomes a thoughtful deed for the simple fact that you agreed to make it part of your commitment. It becomes extra valuable when you stick to that commitment without being prodded, and hopefully, your partner takes notice and responds with gratitude and appreciation.

If it's usually her assignment to cook dinner nightly, then you can end one evening with a thoughtful deed of a massage as a way of expressing your gratitude and appreciation—on top of thoughtful words that also tell her so. Now that will surely tell her that her cooking is doubly valuable in your eyes.

What I would like to emphasize here is that the mood and tone of the actions should feel like expressions of love and romance. If they come off as obligations you had to fulfill, duties you have no choice but to render, or praise-worthy acts you want to show off, you devalue the entire thing. I know of men who do these things but then brag about it in parties or social media, or they grumble while doing them, or they use it to "barter" for reciprocal acts of service from their spouse (I'll mop up the mess, you clean the cat litter). By doing so, it definitely becomes just an "act" of service.

The language of Romance revolves around deeds that aren't only thoughtful but heartfelt too.

C. Kindness: Earlier in this book, I'd cited a study involving 68,000 people that revealed *kindness* as the most desirable trait in a partner by nearly 90% of women surveyed. Aside from that, researchers from

Swansea University in Wales also asked college-aged students from 59 countries to rank the following traits according to what they value the most in an ideal romantic partner: physical attractiveness, desire to have children, chastity, kindness, humor, creativity, religiosity, and good financial prospects. Kindness came out the most important quality across the globe.

There's separate research which likewise indicates that kindness (along with emotional stability) is the key predictor of satisfaction and stability in a marriage. And another nice thing about practicing kindness is that there's a good deal of evidence showing how individuals who receive or witness kindness are more likely to become kind themselves.[25] So you could be leading the two of you into a more loving relationship by sheer example!

Romance is a partnership of hearts. And what people are looking for in that partnership is a sense of comfort and safety. Kindness is the trait that infuses that partnership with a feeling like you're home. It has a quality of selflessness about it as you become considerate and caring of your partner, creating a climate of trust—constantly. *Thoughtful Kindness* doesn't flicker. It's not something that comes and goes. It allows her to have complete faith, day after day, that the last person in the world who would hurt her is you.

Being unkind could be unintentional or habitual for either you or your partner. You or she may not even realize you're being unkind. Such as always needing to be right or being in a bad mood and quick to get angry. It could be a habit of criticizing, contradicting, correcting, flirting with someone else, lying, not apologizing, not thanking. It could show a lack of respect for each other's time if either one of you is constantly late, not responding to texts and calls in a timely manner, and always saying "later." One could be overly suspicious or jealous, not compromising, sharing, or considering what the other prefers or wants.

Our words could also be harsher than we think, such as those backhanded compliments, sarcastic remarks, or subtle digs. This hurts at any time and is magnified tenfold when done to get a laugh from others. Instead of saying his wife looks lovely in her party dress, a man might say, "She cleans up real nice, doesn't she?" Or instead of praising her lasagna, he'd go, "I'd come home early if you cooked like this every day." Sometimes, he might give a smart-alecky answer just to keep from sounding mawkish or mushy or because he doesn't want to look "soft" in front of his friends. Or he might be doing it to let out some bottled-up resentment or as retaliation over some unsettled grievance. Whatever the reason, it is unkind.

Unkind behavior often rears its ugly head as some passive-aggressive means of dealing with conflict. There is a better way to handle your disagreements and bruised emotions, and that will be discussed in the next chapter.

All relationship experts will tell you, it's not the lavish gifts and grand displays that make a relationship stronger. It's the little things spread out throughout your days that build it, brick by sturdy brick. Kindness is as simple as being on time when you're meeting her somewhere. It's drinking the flavor of tea she doesn't like so she can have all of the ones she prefers. It's making the steak well-done for her if that's how she wants it, even if you think it's better medium rare. It's laughing at her jokes, and not laughing at her mistakes. It's being quick in granting requests, answering messages, returning a call. Finding the earliest possible time to do so despite our busy lives underscores her importance. And you do this all out of kindness, not because you're avoiding being nagged. Let it flow out of you, naturally, without waiting for her to sulk or call you out on it. It's looking for opportunities to be nice, supportive, and considerate.

The Thoughtful Action Plan: Reviewed

Our trek has taken us close to the other end of the enchanted forest, and we settle down by a brook lined with fragrant flowers of deep red, white, and yellow gold. Magical flowers, I assume. What else can one expect from an enchanted forest?

As we relax in the calming shade, I give a recap of our Thoughtful Action Plan on how to speak the language of Romance.

Be her FRIEND

• Beyond saying you love her, use **Thoughtful Words** to express your gratitude, appreciation, admiration, support, and encouragement frequently.

• Give **Thoughtful Gifts** that clearly show how much you know her likes and favorites, needs and wants. As the saying goes—more than the price—it's the thought that *really* counts.

• Grant her **Thoughtful Freedom** that allows her to enjoy her family, friends, and community, her private world, her time away for whatever she pleases—with no other reason than for her to feel free.

Be her LOVER

• Give **Thought to your Presentation**. Part of wanting to be a better man for her is wanting to be a better-looking man for her. Aim far beyond being presentable. Be the gift she wants to unwrap.

• Beyond just spending time together in the same room, invest in **Thoughtful Togetherness** which means looking for meaningful ways that bring you closer to each other.

• **Thoughtful Contact** makes touching, kissing, hugging, and looking in each other's eyes intentional and longer-lasting, several times a day. Every day.

Be her PARTNER

• **Thoughtful Attention** is done in response to both her subtle and obvious cues in ways that recognize her personal needs, quirks, and unique desires.

• Perform **Thoughtful Deeds** which are meaningful and heartfelt expressions of love—encompassing both what's expected of you and the things you choose to do beyond that to make life feel a lot lighter.

• Kindness is more than doing nice things for her now and then. **Thoughtful Kindness** is constant. It's giving her faith that you will do everything, at all times, to provide a loving space full of trust, respect, and peace, where she always feels you have her back.

Just as I finish my review of the lessons from this leg of the journey, we hear the galloping of hooves. The prince appears along a forest path, breathless from his dragon-slaying expedition but still looking freshly bathed.

"Greetings, oh merry band of brave-hearted men," he says as his horse skitters to a stop. "How goes your quest?"

"It's going rather well," I say. "I've just finished recounting to them how to be a Prince Charming who keeps on charming—long after courtship is done."

"Long after courtship?" he asks, quirking his brow. "That's poppycock! Everybody knows that after I get the girl, that's where the story ends."

I chuckle. "In the real world, that's where the story begins."

"Pray tell. How is that possible?" He dismounts from his trusty steed. "A prince needs to go back to his princely duties. There are dragons to slay. Oceans to be sailed. New lands to be conquered."

"Yeah, each man here has his own version of that. Can you tell them how you keep charming the girl while you're doing all that?" I ask.

"One cannot!" He thrusts his fists into his hips. "Precisely why that's where the fairy tale ends."

I glance encouragingly at my brigade of Brave Hearts. "Lucky for us, modern real-world research proves it doesn't have to end there."

Can Prince Charming Deal with Two Full-time Jobs?

I'm sure you've heard the phrase, "Love is a verb." You can think of her constantly. You can say "I love you" every day. You can even yearn to be with her every time you're apart. But unless you do enough to show it—consistently—loving her won't mean much at all.

Here's a daunting thought: a long-term romantic relationship should be treated like another full-time job. I realize that most men would probably react to that by saying, "You've got to be sh*tting me!" I believe that attitude is one major reason relationships keep failing. Because most men are raised to believe that career comes first. That the woman is there to support him so he can be the best he can be at his profession or business or mission. And thus, it ends up being a choice: Career vs. Relationship. And quite often, the advice is to prioritize the career, because that is sustainable; it's more within your control; it doesn't come with extra baggage. It defines you.

But does it have to be a choice between Career vs. Relationship? We should realize by now, as superior animals of the Earth with two astounding hemispheres to our brain and an amazing neocortex to boot—we have the capacity to have both. Having a flourishing career and a great relationship is like having two full-time jobs—one superimposed seamlessly over the other.

Love used to be an optional element in marriage. These days, 90% of those who choose to marry cite love as their main reason for doing so. Love has become essential—but it's not enough. There was a time men worked harder at making money than in keeping their wives emotionally satisfied and happy—because those wives stayed no matter what. Usually, because they didn't have a choice. Nowadays, women are working hard to earn money too, and are likewise expected to keep their husbands emotionally and sexually satisfied while keeping the home and family in order. Husbands and wives are both thinking—it's too much hard work.

But if you broke it down into simple hours, it's really not "too much." To be mathematical about it, there are 168 hours in a week, and a regular full-time job typically consumes about 40 hours of that week. If you considered marriage a second full-time job, then subtract another 40 hours from the total, and that still leaves you 88 hours for everything else outside of work and married life. Let's say you sleep six to eight hours a night, that will still leave you roughly another 40 hours just for yourself. If all you devoted to your partner was three hours a week for a date plus one hour for making love, that means you're giving this precious relationship in your life a mere 10% of what your job gets. Not 10% of your total time, but only 10% of what you give your job. Exactly how valuable is this woman to you compared to your boss?

There are couples who've been together for decades who say they are still as in love today as in the early years of their marriage. And they work hard at it!

A successful career coexisting with a satisfying relationship may seem rare. A McKinsey survey found that across the professional sectors, both men and women reported themselves to be happier with their jobs when they were part of a single-career couple.[26] But in the UK where 70% of professionals are working couples, the lowest divorce rate (48% below the baseline) is among couples who earn about the same amount and contribute comparable amounts to household expenses. There's also a growing body of sociological research giving evidence that when both partners dedicate themselves to work *and* to home life, the benefits are far-reaching.[27] It gives the couple more financial freedom, a more satisfying relationship, and a lower-than-average chance of divorce.

The research also indicates that good relationships and career satisfaction don't have to be mutually exclusive. What it takes is deliberate planning and cooperation between partners. Roles can shift as the years go by, and having both parties discuss the corresponding shifts in their share of duties and contributions results in a union where the balance of a fulfilling relationship, satisfying careers, and responsible child-rearing is co-designed, and thus successfully accomplished.

Once again, good communication takes center stage as the key to a strong and lasting romantic partnership. And despite the discouraging statistics surrounding divorce, a growing number of studies have shown that of the marriages that don't break up, a large percentage of couples do in fact stay happy. That includes a 2012 survey of Americans who've been married for ten or more years; it states that 40% of these couples identify themselves as being still "very intensely" in love with their partner.[28] More recently, the 2023 Gitnux Marketdata Report states that 64% of married Americans say they are "very happy" in their relationships. In arranged marriages, which statistically have proven far more stable than "love marriages," the couples report that they start out learning to like their spouse then feel the love grow and get stronger through the years.

Arthur Aron, a social psychologist at Stony Brook University, conducted a study of brain scans from adults in long-term marriages who professed to being as much in love now as they were at the very beginning of their relationship.[29] Aron compared those brain scans with that of couples who had just fallen in love. The result showed similar activity in both types of couples in the reward-processing region of the brain.

"There is actually a possibility that it's not just a fairy tale," Aron says, "that there are people that live happily ever after. Some people actually do it." And these happy couples assert that it takes a lot of hard work.

The moral of the story of Prince Charming? A happy lifelong relationship isn't something you wish upon a star for. We need to work hard at living happily ever after.

The prince, enlightened by the real-world information I shared, motions towards the row of deep red and yellow gold flowers growing by the brook. "Those are everlasting flowers whose beauty never fades." He invites us all to pluck one each to take with us on our quest. "May it inspire you to forever be the Prince Charming in your lady's life."

What Prince Charming, Q, and James Bond Have in Common

A Prince Charming, who keeps on charming, sets the example of a man who keeps the courtship going. He sees no end date to the chase. Even after he's won her heart, put a ring on her finger, exchanged vows, raised a family, and they're now alone together in their empty nest, he still finds delight in delighting her. He *never stops* winning her heart.

Q, Jarvis, and Alfred all recognize the importance of their contributions to make things work so the world doesn't come crashing down on anybody. They *never stop* paying attention and giving their support. And by following their example, you get to ease the brakes in your woman's troubled mind, helping her to relax, and open herself up to you intimately.

James Bond is the man you outdo by treating your high-value lady the way she deserves. With respect and admiration. You *never stop* wanting to bond with her and make her feel valued as a person.

Even though I kept repeating the phrase "never stop," it's not literally a 24/7 thing, done 365 days of the year. Rule No. 2 (Do things that show her you love her) is about being consistent, not incessant.

Billy Crystal's iconic line that "Women need a reason to have sex, men just need a place" paraphrases the warning imprinted at a young age in women's minds, that men are just after one thing. She needs a reason to make love—which explains why you need those three kinds of foreplay. The things you do "In Advance" and "In Her Heart" count a lot, because if all you do is put on the charm just as a last-minute intro to "In the Moment" foreplay, it will work against you in the long run.

This might seem baffling to you. Why would it upset her if you only turn the 'sexy' on when it's time to have sex? What the heck is wrong with that?

Before I lay down the explanation, I'm giving you a heads up that we're only a few steps away from the precious nugget of relationship advice I'd told you I'd buried like a treasure in the middle of this book. So read through the next paragraphs carefully because it leads to that rare gem.

What PET Scans Reveal

The answer as to why women believe men never listen, forget everything, and don't seem to care what women feel and think goes back to the differences in how the male and female brains are hard-wired. Our pre-historic examples Drrahd and Kro-ah illustrated how men and women have always differed in how they needed to function. PET scans of modern men and women show the underlying differences are still very much there despite the tremendous changes in societal structures and cultural expectations.[30] PET scans allow us to see colors lighting up in the brain, giving us a dynamic, real-time illustration of male-female differences in living color. The sections that light up tell us which parts of the brain are more engaged or recruited to perform a particular task.

To this day, men's brains require less involvement from the emotive centers and memory storage areas when looking at a sad face. (Because as a hunter, he never needed to feel sorry for the bison he was about to kill or maintain a feeling of sadness and/or guilt for leaving behind his wife and kids and all the needs and wants of the people in the tribe. A woman, even though she also hunted, stayed closer to home due to her motherly and other duties.) Men also have more cortical areas devoted to spatial reasoning and fewer verbal centers. Research shows that, on average, men only speak 12,000 words per day compared to women who speak 25,000. (I suppose a group of chattering hunters with poor depth perception wouldn't have had much success.)

To be more task-focused, it became more efficient for the male brain to compartmentalize. In other words, it's natural for men to package life into neat boxes, each one holding its own set of priorities, plans, memories, and so on. This box is for work. This is for my office buddies.

This is for my golf buddies. This box is for chores. This is for my family. This one is for sex.

Imagine the male mind, therefore, as resembling a container warehouse that is organized for efficiency—a place for everything and with everything in its place, allowing him to deal with each important matter one at a time, when he's ready for it.

Women's brains, in comparison, are as colorful as flowering vines that interlace with other vines sprawling over the garden of their lives. PET scans show more colors lighting it up, revealing that the female brain has more nerve connections. Consequently, there's about 15% more blood flow feeding the female brain that constantly cross-signals. Women tend to see more, feel more, and take in more overall. Studies also show they have better memory[31] and as previously mentioned, they talk more too. That's because rather than boxing up their lives, women (and as a result, so did their pre-historic tribes) thrive on making connections and talking things through.

Oftentimes, men stuff their strongest feelings into one steel-reinforced box of its own. Which is rather unfortunate, because that also allows him to isolate his guilt over his indiscretions, so that when he says, "it didn't mean anything," he means it. However, it truly can never be discounted as meaningless by a woman whose emotions are tightly wound with every thought and action that she makes. A flowering vine of a mind simply cannot fathom the compartmentalized nature of a mind full of boxes. She puts meaning in everything. Even in your silence. So that when she asks, "What are you thinking about?" and you say, "Nothing." She still thinks that means something.

Some men are surprised to hear that women don't think in boxes too. I've had a male client exclaim, "How can they not?" with eyes flaring wide as he tried to wrap his head around any other way of thinking. I've had a woman suspect her husband had adult ADHD because she couldn't fathom how he could forget even very important things (because his thoughts were stuck inside a mental box). If you'd like to go deeper into the topic, you can Google "men compartmentalize" to get more information about it. It would be good if men and women alike did so, because not understanding this fundamental difference is at the root of many of our troubles in our relationships.

We weren't seriously taught to expect this kind of disparity in how we deal with everyday life. We can all plainly see there's a difference, of course, but we had to guess at the explanation, sometimes going as far as blaming patriarchy, radical feminism, or toxic masculinity for *every* little disappointment. We need to hear something as basic as biology and neurochemistry, explained with the objective tone of a researcher or science teacher laying down the facts. Yes, upbringing and culture play a part in the adults we turn out to be, but a huge bulk of who we are is beyond our ability to override. A woman cannot nag and cold-shoulder a man into lowering his sex drive. (He may, instead, learn to conceal it and find some other release.) A man cannot yell and punch a woman into not noticing everything he forgot. (She may stop pointing them out, but her brain will still notice.) Even before we are born—weeks into gestation—the differences are already there. Not knowing and/or acknowledging this fact has deprived us of the ability to be more accepting, forgiving, and appreciative of our contrasting-yet-complementary natures.

Sadly, therefore, we grew up with our male-female differences discussed with bitter sarcasm by one gender representative versus the other. "Men!" women exclaim with a roll of their eyes. "Women," men groan with a pinch of their brows.

Which is why your partner is likely to get upset when you don't text her in the middle of your workday to say you miss her, because it tells her all you were thinking about was work. And which is why you get frustrated when you just want to sprawl on the couch and focus on a game on TV while she rants about her day then tosses in a request for you to check the flickering light bulb in the hallway then sneaks in a quick kiss and thank you—none of which register because there was a jaw-dropping three-point shot that happened around that time.

With this simple declaration, I can now say—

X

marks the spot

Yes, we've come to the buried treasure at the center of this book: my promised answer to the question, "What does a woman want?"

It all boils down to the container warehouse in your compartmentalized head.

REVELATION: WHAT DOES A WOMAN WANT?

HAVE A LOOK AT how you've organized the boxes that organize your days. Take an inventory of it. List down the contents of each of the compartments and give them a name. For example, you can name one box "Business" or "Job." If you have both, then that's two compartments right there. List down all the elements of your life that complete the entire you, each one taking its share of your time, energy, and thoughts. These could include Running, Jiu Jitsu, Social media, Drinking nights, Household chores, Pets, Travel, Gaming, Sex, etc.

Finally, I'm about to tell you what your partner wants, and I'm warning you upfront, it's not something you can give.

She wants you to put her inside each one of those compartments. It's like having you drill holes into every box inside your head so you can slip thoughts and feelings about her into every one of them. Whether it's during overtime work, your golf game, your Friday night out, your trip to the barber, while you're watching porn. What that means is, she's looking for signs from you that she doesn't completely leave your mind night or day, whatever it is you're doing (after all, thoughts of random things related to you linger in her mind day and night).

It's not that she literally *wants* it from you, but that's how she functions. It's like she's responding to a subconscious alarm that goes off when her partner doesn't exhibit signs he's thinking about her as much as she's thinking about him, implying she's been forgotten. So, it concerns her. Maybe even upsets her. Eventually, it could anger her. Mainly because she doesn't know that the biological difference between your brain and hers is the reason you didn't text her in the middle of a conference, or didn't advise her you'd be late for dinner, and that you even forgot you agreed to attend your kid's recital.

These could all be attributed to your brain being stuck in one compartment, and you weren't able to shift your focus in time. Because of that, she takes it personally. It feels like you didn't care or you're not trying hard enough. She thinks that, if you remember everything you need to do at work, then why couldn't you remember to buy the milk she asked for on your way home? The answer, simply put, is because you were thinking about work while working and about driving while driving. Or maybe, while driving, your brain went on autopilot, so you switched to thinking about nothing. And by nothing, you mean nothing. But to her, that means you should have remembered she had asked for something.

I hope by now you've gained some clarity as to why you're running as fast as you can, but she still thinks you're not running fast enough. And it seems like the only way you can keep up with her expectations is to drill holes in your brain so colorful flowering vines can grow through your gray matter. That, or divorce.

Take a deep breath. There's no need for either radical measure, because I have a more feasible suggestion that I believe men in happy, long-term relationships have already been doing.

Do this, and you'll see a remarkable change in your relationship too: Give her a compartment with her name on it.

Hats off to you if you already had that on your list of compartments. And by *her name*, I mean that of the woman at her core who isn't playing any roles of wife or girlfriend or mother or housemate or lover. When she's just being herself for herself.

I know of men who can rattle off trivia about all the aircraft featured in the *Top Gun* movies. Or name nearly every single character in the *Star Wars* saga and talk about their backgrounds. Or discuss movie directors both famous and obscure and what's great about each one of them. But ask them about their wives, and they would have no idea what her happiest childhood memory is. Or her saddest. Or what career she would rather have if she weren't doing what she was doing now.

Check inside the box where you plan to put her name and take out all the items related to the kids and family life, religion, housework, errands, sex, entertainment, vacations—because all these already have their separate boxes.

All you should have left inside is time, energy, and thoughts devoted only to her, just her, and purely her. (You probably had that box during courtship, but dust has since covered up her name.) This box should be filled with truths about the inner her that you've gathered while you were connecting warmly with her, and you weren't arguing, eating, drinking, texting, scrolling, playing, watching, or engaged in any other activity. It should be that part of her that also had no other activities or people or concerns on her mind while interacting with you. No planning, no packing, no watching over anyone, worrying about anything, no fighting, or pleasing anyone.

In short, it's a box containing stuff she would only share with the people closest to her. Or, more importantly, they're things only someone as special as you would ever know.

That box will also hold precious memories she holds of you. All the things only you would give to her, deeds that have become extra meaningful because they came from you. Such as you, focusing on her stories about her achievement at work and taking out a bottle of champagne for a toast just between the two of you. You, canceling a road trip with your buddies because she's had a major upset, and she needs your emotional support. You, telling her how beautiful she is, when all she sees in the mirror are her wrinkles and graying hair. You, surprising her with a little quirky thing that you know for sure she would love—because you know her that well and that deeply.

That. That is the box with her name on it. How much is in it? Is the box worthy of being wrapped with a giant bow on top? If not, and you'd like to fill it up so she can feel you don't need flowery vines to stay connected to her, read on about Rule No. 3.

5

Rule No. 3: Feel Your Feelings and Soften Them Up

THERE'S A SCENE IN the movie *Avengers: Infinity War* wherein Thor's hammer, the Stormbreaker, has been shattered. For it to be reforged, Thor needs to use all his godly might to hold open the iris of the forge and take on the full force of a neutron star so its power can be harnessed. He braces himself at the center of the iris then roars in agony as the blazing inferno blasts through it, searing his flesh, nearly killing him. In the end, it's the Stormbreaker itself, fully restored, that saves his life.

It's a gripping scene—and it was the first image that came to mind when I was thinking of a metaphor for what it feels like for a man dealing with an onslaught of emotions. Why? Because I imagine that the default state of a man's "iris" or doorway to his emotions is shut, and it takes Herculean effort (or should I say, Thor-ian effort) to hold it open for the opposite sex.

It might seem like equating a talk with your partner with the god of thunder enduring the concentrated energy of a neutron star is an exaggeration. It would be—if she were a gem who stayed level-headed even during an argument. But sometimes, a woman raging and shouting and hurling objects in anger at a man could feel like the mighty Thor allowing himself to be overpowered by thunder.

If the only thing a man and a woman were to talk about was the Marvel universe, what his favorite movie was, or if he thought Loki was a good or bad guy—then that's easy-peasy. But once it strays into, "Why do you always forget the things I say?" Or, "I'm bothered by how much you still talk with your mother." Or, "I'm not comfortable with how you handled that incident with the kids."

Time and again, men say how draining it is when a woman wants to "have a talk." And it's not even because there's an argument going on. Simply allowing feelings to flow in and out while staying focused on and attuned to the woman so he can give the appropriate responses, sucks the life force out of him.

In the movie, Thor had to hold the iris open for less than a minute. How long can you hold the iris to your heart open before crumbling in exhaustion?

What I'm aiming to address in this section are those situations when the woman's ire is driven by her inability to connect with a man's emotions. When getting him to feel what she's feeling seems impossible because of an impenetrable wall or a huge distance between them. So she turns to anger or some other release of her frustration as a way to get a response from a man who stays emotionally unavailable despite her attempts to connect.

Letting feelings flow is tough for a man to do because of his biology, bolstered by a lifetime of programming that told him all things emotional are for girls, gays, and goofballs. There are men who even have to re-learn how to cry after training themselves to hold back their tears since childhood. Hardly anyone tells a young boy that being attuned and responsive to someone else's feelings, as well as his own, are part of being a gentleman. Oftentimes, even just identifying what he's feeling in a certain moment is beyond him. Men are familiar with anger and disgust, as well as certain levels of sadness and joy. But he needs to stifle showing fear, shame or guilt. Sometimes even surprise (heaven forbid that he lets out a shriek). And worst of all, love.

For a man to be more in touch and honest about his feelings: There was a time when I wondered if it was even fair of women to ask this of men. After all, it entails battling against both his biological nature and cultural programming to be open about what he feels—even to himself! This stifling of emotions was built in for the survival of the species and reinforced for the formation and protection of nations. And now, in the modern era, men need to go against that if they want to keep their romantic relationships intact. Because now, women can walk away.

But then I looked at the flipside of the coin.

For a woman to be more open, adventurous, and giving of herself when it comes to sex: This is the unspoken wish a man may find very difficult, if not impossible, to express to his significant other. I'm not speaking of a woman still in the dating game or in the early stages of a relationship where hormonal cocktails are flooding her system. I'm talking about a woman in a long-term commitment where the man's shining armor has begun to dull in her eyes. Where his charm no longer works like it used to. When the rose tint on the lenses through which she saw him has turned blue. That's when thinking about him only adds to the long list of things she needs to do.

We've already discussed how making love, for her, entails complete cooperation of her brain, and that she has to be emotionally connected for her to truly find pleasure in it. We've also gone through the statistics of how elusive orgasms could be for many women, which means she can go through the motions without really "feeling" it.

Based on a comprehensive review of 150 studies, social psychologist Roy F. Baumeister et al. concluded that the male sex drive is most definitely stronger.[32] Their paper states, "Across many different studies and measures, men have been shown to have more frequent and more intense sexual desires than women, as reflected in spontaneous thoughts about sex, frequency and variety of sexual fantasies, desired frequency of intercourse, desired number of partners, masturbation, liking for various sexual practices, willingness to forego sex, initiating versus refusing sex, making sacrifices for sex, and other measures." In addition, they found no evidence to the contrary, meaning there was nothing that would indicate stronger sexual motivation among women.

I suppose many will think we don't need a study to confirm this. It's been said many times before that "men only want one thing." But what is seldom heard is that men consider sex as a means to connect and deepen intimacy when they're with someone they love. For him, he's literally *making* love. The act of sex helps create the emotional bond for him. Whereas with women, the emotional bond needs to be there first.

What this tells you is that there is an imbalance that could lead to a vicious cycle of unmet needs. Women want men to be more emotionally vulnerable so they can feel more sexual desire. Men want women to be sexually available so they can be more comfortable being vulnerable. Yet both sides find it challenging to deliver what is expected of them.

Which is why I've come to the conclusion that it's only fair that men push themselves to become emotionally open, in much the same way that women should make themselves more welcoming of sexual intimacy—because these needs feed off each other. It's like a symbiosis of sorts.

I realize some people might bristle over that suggestion and say that a woman has come a long way from when her sole ambition was to marry and have children, lived in fear that her husband would die, come home crippled, or leave her. And so, all he had to do was come home alive and well, and she'd be happy (provided he was a good man who didn't beat her up). She'd remain grateful till the end of her days that he had chosen to marry her (or agreed to, because most marriages were arranged back then), sparing her the stigma of becoming an old maid and dying childless. A woman used to have to pay her debt of gratitude every single day; she cooked, cleaned, cared for the children, and let him "bed" her *regardless of how she felt*.

"Not anymore, mister!" would be today's collective cry.

Well, now that we've gone through the earlier parts of this book, both sides should now be capable of seeing things in a different light. So let's reframe the situation.

Reframing is a technique used by psychotherapists to help people shift their mindset. Think of a frame as the context through which you view a situation, person, or a relationship. Changing the "frame" means letting yourself see things from a new perspective. When you reframe it, it could turn something previously seen as negative into something neutral or even positive.

Say for instance that whenever you initiated sex, your wife might have thought, "He's so inconsiderate. I'm so tired and stressed, and all he can think about is gratifying himself." That's when all she believes is that sex is nothing but a strong biological need for you—and she doesn't know about that entire compartment in your heart and mind dedicated to her. In that box with her name on it, sex is part of communicating deeply with her and is a very important means by which you connect with her, enabling you to become emotionally vulnerable. If she comes to realize that making love with her is something you need so you can share and immerse in that love, then hopefully, she will reframe it and see it as something you need *for the both of you*.

In turn, whenever she starts to talk about her feelings and wants to know yours, or when she asks for more time with you, or keeps pointing out how you weren't paying attention to her—you might have always thought, "She's so controlling. I'm not her kid. Why am I always wrong?" But now, you know that she couldn't relate to that system you have of containers in your head. That it doesn't make sense how you can love her and yet forget about her while you're doing other things. That she couldn't understand how not remembering the things she said and that your need for "me time" doesn't mean you love her less.

When you've come to realize that she's not blaming you and is only looking after the village in her head, then you can reframe each situation and see that what she needs are constant signals from you that say *she really is on your mind*. And you do that by filling up that compartment with her name on it with meaningful moments that touch her heart.

You can only manage that by opening up your heart to her.

A Disclaimer on Her Wishes

I do need to point out a gnarl in the fabric here. There are women who constantly say they wish their partner could be more open about their feelings, but when it happens, they end up shaming him for acting like a wuss. "Don't be such a baby," she'd say, if he breaks into tears over his blunder or failure, then she pushes him back to the tough role where she feels more comfortable seeing him. "Be the man. You've got this."

Quite unfairly, she may simply be wishing that he be more open to *her* feelings, whereas she remains unprepared for his.

This brings us back to Rule No. 1: Know who you love, and why. Is she someone you can trust with your heart when you find the courage to let her in? I have seen beautiful relationships where the man can reveal his childish, irrational fears and the woman remains fully supportive and compassionate, knowing that every person has an Achilles' heel. I sincerely hope that you've found an emotionally stable and mature woman who can and will support you when you're down. She needs to understand your need for a soft place to land.

Of course, there is a limit to what a partner can tolerate or accept. There is a right balance to a man's emotional strength and vulnerability, just as there is with hers—when her sense of independence and empowerment can go beyond admirable and become overbearing. Many men and women are still teetering on their toes, often unsure where that balance lies given all the old-world programming they've received since childhood. There's a lot of reprogramming and calibration that's still being done on either side.

Don't be The Hulk. Don't give in to anger.

Rule No. 3: Feel Your Feelings and Soften Them Up

Our next stop is a small cabin in the wilderness. A perfect hideaway for a man who wants to steer clear of anything that could rile him.

"Are you ready to meet The Hulk?" I ask as we march up the pathway leading to the porch.

"That would be incredible," you say with a smirk.

I snort out a chuckle. "Seriously. Now's the time to think of anything you'd like to ask him."

You scratch your head. "Do we really want to get into a conversation with an angry guy?"

"Of course not." I knock on the cabin door. "There's no talking with an angry guy."

A few seconds later, a disheveled though amiable-looking fellow welcomes our party into his quiet refuge. It's Dr. Bruce Banner, the mild-mannered scientist, physicist, and medical doctor whose seven

PhDs and profound intellect are no match for his rage when he turns into the Incredible Hulk.

"Would you like some coffee?" he asks in a pleasant, calm tone.

We all accept the offer, and he places a good old-fashioned kettle on the traditional stove. He invites us all to have a seat as we wait for the water to boil.

Bruce Banner's character has a famous line. "Don't make me angry. You wouldn't like me when I'm angry." Eventually, Banner had revealed his secret: "I'm always angry."

I believe those are words many men don't realize are lurking in their subconscious. In his book *The Macho Paradox*, author Jackson Katz wrote that, "Countless men deal with their vulnerability by transferring vulnerable feelings to feelings of anger. The anger then serves to 'prove' that they are not, in fact, vulnerable, which would imply they are not man enough to take the pressure."

This means anger, like The Hulk, can be a mask that hides a vulnerable man underneath. A man who lashes out at his wife, who'd been talking for hours with her friends, might be hiding his fear that she finds his company boring. When he blows his top because she's taking too long prettying herself up for a party, he might be concealing a fear that she's out to attract another man. When he flies off the handle because she keeps correcting him, he might be fighting his fear that she thinks he's not smart enough.

Several times, I've mentioned that a man is often a stranger to his own feelings. That makes it far more difficult for him to be able to express himself eloquently to his partner at a time of conflict. This then leads to a tendency to avoid tough conversations altogether. I'd mentioned earlier that fighting wasn't something I went through in my marriage. We had stilted conversations leaving behind decades-worth of unresolved issues—which inevitably led to the end of our marriage. So avoiding disagreements is not the solution either; it just buries the problem until it takes root and turns into an ugly, gnarled, thorny growth that destroys the foundation of your commitment.

At the other end of the spectrum is having too many arguments, too much fighting, which happens to be one of the leading causes of divorce. Quite likely, even if she'd gone all-out irrational, hurling objects and expletives at him, a gentleman would just curl his hands into fists, hold his anger in, and then storm off, putting up a thick stone wall of silence. (Do note that a woman who gets out of control and demonstrates no respect for you—despite you staying on the reasonable side of the fence—might have issues that could spring from childhood trauma, neglect, abandonment, or abuse. If so, those are things she would need help with from a counselor or therapist in order to uncover and heal.)

This section of the book is to help you stay in that healthy in-between zone where you face conflicts head on and deal with them in a constructive way, where you can talk with each other and disagree without letting anger take over.

There are situations, of course, which warrant anger as the response. When someone threatens you or any of your loved ones—then anger will spark beyond your control. But when it comes to romantic relationships, there are healthier, more productive ways of dealing with conflict. You deserve to have your needs met, and so does she. In the next few pages, I'll be giving suggestions on how to handle disagreements, establish boundaries, and resolve conflicts while keeping anger out of the room.

I must admit, these are lessons I had to seek out and learn a little too late. One major misconception I had when I entered my marriage was that happy couples fight less—or don't fight at all. That's because I grew up not ever seeing my parents fight, at least not until after they told us they were separating. So my juvenile mind concluded that having arguments equals a marriage falling apart.

In reality, though, psychology experts who've studied relationships for decades have concluded that happy couples do argue.[33] Quite a lot, sometimes. But the big difference is that they argue productively. They don't argue just to vent or to attack. They face the issue together, so it's not about you vs. me. It becomes us vs. the problem.

And that's the key element here. That you are both good partners (remember the roles we discussed in the previous chapter? You as friend, lover, and *partner*). It means both of you extend kindness to one another and are respectful of each other's boundaries. If one or both of you are too self-centered or are unable to empathize with the other (such as those with a dark personality trait) then even the best communication skills during a moment of conflict may prove futile.

With that said, I hope to make it clear that learning to handle conflicts better can lead to one of two things: it can enhance your relationship and make it stronger, or it could show you that your differences are irreconcilable and that it would be better for you to move on. Either way, it should lead you to a happier life.

Here's my simple suggestion. The next time you feel that she's driving you nuts with her behavior or is driving you up the wall with her attitude: Drive a BeMW.

Is She Driving You Crazy? Think BMW.

Conflicts are such difficult, exhausting, and inescapable things that even the happiest of marriages go through. I've made the following technique and its explanation as straightforward as I can to make conflict resolution less daunting.

In the heat of an argument, it may be difficult to remember complex tips, so I came up with this acronym: BeMW—pronounced like the famous car brand. It's to help you slam your foot on the brakes, giving you time to recall the three steps you need to take when you find yourself about to drive headlong into conflict.

The next time you feel slighted, think BeMW before you respond.

B – Behavior: State her behavior that has upset you

eM – Emotion: Name the emotion the behavior triggered in you

W – Wish: State what you wish she would do next time

For example, you've just come home after a tiring day at work, and the first thing she does is complain about how you left your wet towel on the bed that morning. The first feeling you'd probably have is annoyance or irritation, which are derivations or permutations of anger. Dig deeper and ask yourself why you're mad. What nerve did she hit? Figure that out and you may be able to identify the feelings hiding behind your anger.

If you can't put your finger on exactly what your secondary emotions are, rein in your impulse to lash out at her and instead, ask for a few minutes so you can first wind down then discuss. You were probably hurt when she called you out on that wet towel because she didn't consider the fact you were running late, even though she knew you had an important meeting first thing. You'd much prefer it if she just gave you a gentle reminder about it and expressed some understanding.

After you've gotten a better hold of yourself, you can then pick up the conversation and say, "When I came home from work and the first thing I got was a reprimand for leaving that wet towel (*point out the behavior matter-of-factly with no accusation; also avoiding the accusatory word "you"*), I felt hurt (*name your feeling; use "I felt" or "I feel" depending on the circumstance*) because I was rushing for an important meeting, that's why it happened. I wish next time, you'd greet me first and extend some understanding after a long hard day (*state your wish*). You can mention the wet towel later."

It's difficult for most people—male or female—to identify the emotion that was triggered by the behavior, so take some extra time to identify it. Without doing so, you might end up stating your *interpretation* of an action rather than a feeling. For instance, you might say, "I felt attacked," which is your conclusion about her intent. Or you might say, "It felt like your needs matter more than mine," which again is an interpretation of an action rather than a feeling.

By taking extra care to examine the incident, the BeMW sequence helps you skip accusing or blaming. Because stating a behavior as a plainly observed action makes it a non-accusing statement of fact. So be specific. Avoid generalizing. Don't say "You always interrupt." "You never agree." Say instead, "When I was telling a story and you cut in to correct me ..." That's a fact. Not an accusation as in, "When I was telling a story and you butted in and made me look foolish..." That's not a fact. That's already a negative interpretation made by you.

To complete the BeMW sequence properly here would be:

B - When I was telling a story and you cut in to correct me ...

eM – *I felt* belittled, and *I felt* foolish because my mistake was called out in front of everyone.

W – I wish you'd just let me finish then correct me in private, so next time, I'll know better.

Making a Sincere Apology

Let's go back to the wet towel incident.

If, on the other hand, leaving that wet towel was really a careless oversight, because you weren't rushing for anything and it's really a bad habit of yours that needs correcting, then that calls for an apology. In which case, the BeMW becomes this:

B – Behavior: State your behavior that had upset her

eM – Emotion: Name the emotion the behavior triggered in her

W – What she wishes you would do: What will you do to fulfill her wish to keep it from happening again

As in the previous instance, hold back the urge to answer her in anger for having pointed out your oversight. The immediate thing you can do is *reframe*—see things from her perspective—then paraphrase everything she'd said and repeat it back to her. It reassures her that you were listening when you're able to say, "I understand you're upset because I left a wet towel on the bed again this morning. I know you're tired of reminding me about it." Then ask for a bit of time to wind down so you can gather your thoughts. You'll probably really need that time, because it will be more of a challenge for you to name the emotion behind *her* anger.

After you've pondered the situation, you can bring it up again after both of you have cooled your tempers and you can say: "I'm sorry for leaving another wet towel on the bed (*specify the behavior you're apologizing for*). I realize it makes you feel ignored (*name her feeling*) because you've reminded me about that several times before. I can get a small hamper and place it by my side of the bed (*state what you will do to keep it from happening again*) so it will help me remember not to do it again."

A few important things that will make this a great apology.

1. You're not going to justify what you did – "But you know how forgetful I am. You should know that by now."

2. You're not going to accuse her of something right back – "You sometimes forget to wash your coffee cup in the morning. Do I complain?"

3. You're not going to blame her for your actions – "Well, if you didn't keep reminding me I was running late, I wouldn't have left it there."

4. You're not going to tell her she shouldn't feel what she's feeling – "You have no reason to be upset. It's not like the mattress is ruined, is it?"

5. You're not going to bring up the past. – "Did I get on your case when you kept forgetting to put the car keys where they belong?"

6. You're not going to promise it won't happen again, because if it does, she'll just be more disappointed. Fulfill her wish instead. – "I promise to get that hamper this weekend." (And make sure you do it.)

When the Water Boils

I've shared a lot about anger with Bruce Banner listening in, and by this time, we all have steaming cups of coffee in our hands. Our host has taken a seat on a tall stool across from us, with his own mug in hand.

"May I ask a question?" you say, and Banner nods as he takes a sip of hot coffee.

"I've been in that situation a few times when she says something absolutely annoying, and I just ..." You shrug. "How do you not just give in to the anger?"

Banner rubs his stubbled jaw in thought then glances at his stove. "Do you know it can take as little as two minutes for a cup of water to boil in a small pot over high heat at sea level?" He glances around at our group. "A lot of conditions need to be in place for things to get to a rolling boil that fast. So when you feel that hot temper flare ..." He looks straight at you. "Remember to pause."

Sound advice. And I realize it could be difficult to hold back your impulse to just flare up right there and then. But Brave Hearts find the strength to fight the urge and take a pause to give themselves the chance to *reframe*. Seeing the situation only from your perspective will most likely show that you have every right to be upset—and that she's being unreasonable. Change the point of view and look at it through her eyes, reframe, and feel what she feels. Maybe she's angry on the surface, but beneath that, she could be feeling either neglected, jealous, disregarded, disrespected, misunderstood, forgotten, or any other feeling besides simply angry.

This pause that you take ... That break you ask for before you speak up so you can ponder and reframe the situation. It gives you time to look inside yourself. Is this really you reacting—or some younger version of yourself feeling attacked in a hidden memory from your past. What about her? Is this the present-day her? Or a different her dealing with a childhood pain? Is this argument really about today or a new expression of an old, recurring theme?

That pause that you take ... can also be repeated in the heat of an argument. If you did your best to begin the conversation calmly, but emotions erupted anyway, then take a break. Create a conflict "circuit breaker" that will keep either of you from blowing a fuse. It could be a touch or a soft embrace, a phrase (Hey, I'm here for you), a gesture (a hand over your heart), a joke (I think I just farted out my frustration), or a signal (hands forming a T to signal a timeout). That circuit breaker can be a very private thing for couples. Like a code word or safe phrase you both agree on, like "let's chill." It's something that puts a pause to a fight before emotions short circuit, and it allows you to come back to the talk a lot calmer. Find what works for you.

This ability to pause ... and hold your anger at bay. This is what sets you apart from couples in our pre-historic past like Drrahd and Kro-ah whose only concern was survival. Constantly being in an attack-and-defend mode was acceptable, and quite likely expected among men of that era. Romance, thoughtfulness, kindness? Those would have been irrelevant, impractical, and frivolous in the context of their fight for survival. Those qualities in a relationship might have been appreciated—but they were far from imperative. Not like they are now. Back then, a man and woman needed to be strong to stay in loveless relationships. In modern times, they can both be strong enough to walk away. For relationships to become long-term these days, we need to feel loved.

Establishing Boundaries

Now, let's talk about how the BeMW system can help with keeping your boundaries.

"What does that mean exactly anyway?" someone in our group asks. "Setting boundaries. I don't get it."

Bruce Banner offers an explanation. "In a simple sentence, setting a boundary is a pact you make with yourself. You draw a line in the ground, and when someone crosses it—"

"You get angry?" you ask.

"Hopefully not," Banner answers with a subtle smile. "If they cross the line, then I take a course of action that I've decided on before and stick to it."

"For example?" I ask.

"For example, if you hit me when we argue, then I'll move out and stay in a cabin in the wilderness until you get therapy."

"Why would anyone dare to hit you?" someone asks. "Don't they realize what that'll do?"

Banner nods. "That's why they need therapy."

"And that's why you need to make others aware of *your* boundaries," I say. "So they know when they've crossed a line."

We all have this invisible bubble we have around ourselves that we consider our personal space. When someone steps too close, particularly strangers, we feel a boundary has been crossed. Similarly, we have the same invisible boundaries around different aspects of our lives.

For instance, we can accept having our partner poke fun at us, but only so far. We can allow her to have access to our personal possessions, but only so far. We want to be there to help her solve her problems, but only so much. There's a boundary to how far, how much, how often we are willing to allow others to enter our "space" in its various forms and dimensions.

Ideally, if you've become the best of friends, then you already know the lines both of you shouldn't cross to keep the trust going in your relationship. Topics such as money matters, monogamy, sexual expectations, dealing with in-laws, exes, and a host of other things. If there were topics you hadn't discussed before and a boundary suddenly gets crossed, then this is where the BeMW model could come in handy. Though the crossing of boundaries can happen from either direction—because there will certainly be times when you'll push her buttons a little too much— in this book, we'll be looking at things mainly from your side of the story. The principles, however, will be applicable to both sides.

When a boundary of yours has been crossed, point it out to your partner at an opportune time. Think BeMW. Be specific yet matter-of-fact about the behavior that has triggered the sense of resentment, name the ill feelings it has caused without accusing her of ill-intent, and then state your wish regarding the matter. For instance, the boundary that her parents crossed when they expected you both to be at a holiday get-together and your partner simply acquiesced—without regard for your own family's plans. Let's assume that when you started to argue about what happened, you flicked the circuit breaker and did the brave act of fighting your urge to escalate things to a higher level. You stepped back and signaled for a time out (which is different from just storming out then stonewalling). This "time out" means you will resume the discussion. Hopefully, she took your cue and agreed. Then you can pick things up later by saying:

B – When I wasn't consulted about going to that holiday celebration that falls exactly the same time as when my family is having a party—

eM – it made me angry, but also, I felt helpless because you know I wouldn't want to offend your parents. And I also felt hurt and disappointed that my family's plans weren't taken into account. (Being honest about your feelings is a brave act of vulnerability that sidesteps accusing her. Compare that to, "When you and your parents walked all over my family's plans like that, what did you expect? That I'll just go along and not say a thing?")

W – I wish you'd talk to me first before committing to anything for both of us. And I'd rather you give your parents our decision on our behalf, instead of me being put on the spot.

Hopefully, you won't need to confront this issue more than once. If it keeps on happening, then there should be a limit to how many times she can repeatedly cross that same boundary. And the consequence of that is something you need to hold true for yourself.

"You mean, I can threaten to move to a cabin in the wilderness, too, until she gets a new set of parents?" somebody quips.

Banner chuckles. "I'm giving you the benefit of the doubt that the consequences you set will be sensible and fair. That's why you need to think about your boundaries ahead of time. It's a pact you make with your *reasonable* self: if she does this, then I do this. Because Bruce Banner is the one with all the PhDs. The Hulk can't even form a proper sentence. Bruce would say, 'If she hits me, then I call a time out and walk away,' so the Hulk never even makes an appearance. Because the Hulk will definitely do something Bruce will end up regretting."

"Just like I said earlier," I say, "there's no talking to an angry guy."

"What if," you ask, "despite applying the 'reasonable consequence,' she still refuses to change or adjust?"

"Then you need to be prepared to make a decision," I say.

Sometimes, that might mean asking for outside help, like a couples therapist. Or it could mean accepting that the relationship is broken beyond repair and the best decision is to walk away for good. You might be tolerating an unhealthy relationship for fear of ending up alone. Or you're afraid of what others will say. Studies show that people in toxic relationships have a higher chance of suffering heart attacks, strokes, depression, and cancer. Stay in a relationship and fight for it for the right reasons. Your health—and life—depend on it.

This BeMW system can work wonders with conflict resolution if your significant other also embraces the guidelines. You'd be hard-pressed to keep the discussion free of blaming, shaming, and name-calling if she's hell-bent on venting and attacking. She needs to stop seeing you as an issue that needs to be fixed, but rather see the issues as something both of you—as partners—can solve. For this to work, she needs to be a partner in every sense of the word. My hope is that you are in a relationship with a woman secure enough in herself to be able to meet you halfway.

Steering Away from Negativity

Conflict may be unavoidable, but it can be minimized. Keep in mind the number one quality people look for in romantic relationships: Kindness. And the USPs my students had identified for men and women: romance and a soft and safe space, respectively.

Putting those together with other similar findings related to lasting love, it's clear that people are looking for romantic relationships that bring peace to their souls. And yet, these same people find themselves constantly creating a negative dynamic in their desire to create the "perfect" relationship.

Let's refrain from trying to "fix" or "repair" our partners and let them feel loved and accepted for who they are. Know who you love and why. Remember the reason why we are in each other's lives. It's not called a romantic relationship for nothing. We're more than just housemates or chore buddies or constant companions. We're Brave Hearts. Here to do the hard work of making love last.

A huge part of that work is steering clear of the negative triggers. Rather than complaining and criticizing every time we're upset, we can instead express appreciation and gratitude whenever we are pleased. Rather than exploding with anger when we sense disharmony, we can talk things through calmly and you get to understand each other better. Rather than talking about everything bad that's going on in the world, focus on the good things that you have or would like to experience together. Rather than keeping score about who "won" or who got their way the last time, we can let go of our egos and allow the other person to be right.

Social scientist Ty Tashiro shares his research finding in his book *The Science of Happily Ever After: What Really Matters in the Quest for Enduring Love.* He concludes that the top personality trait which best predicts a happy, lifelong partnership is emotional stability.[34] In essence, it's something found in a partner with a positive outlook and who can regulate their emotions. Something Bruce Banner has learned to do on a daily basis.

"I wish you men luck on your hero's journey," Banner says as he leads us to the door. "I try to stay isolated because that's the only way I can find peace. And isolating yourself doesn't have to be in a cabin in the middle of nowhere. It can mean losing yourself in everything else in your life—except your relationship, which is exactly where you *should* be retreating to find peace."

As we all shuffle out, you ask, "Uhm, aren't we going to get a souvenir or something?"

"Souvenir?" Banner asks.

I explain that we have this Knapsack of Knowledge and how those whom we've encountered on the journey have given us something to remind us of lessons learned.

"Oh." Banner looks flustered as he glances back into his barely-furnished cabin.

"How about the mugs?" someone suggests. "To remind us of boiling water."

"How about a BMW?" someone else quips.

Banner blinks. "Tony Stark gave me one." He taps his trouser pockets, as though feeling for keys. "I think I can give you ..."

We all exchange wide-eyed glances.

Banner strides back into the cabin, searches around a work desk, and comes back out to hand you a BMW keychain. "I'm afraid I only have one, but I can send you more."

"Oh, don't worry about it," I say. "I can take care of that. Thank you. It's a perfect reminder of the lessons learned here today."

"Remember to step on the brakes," Banner says. "Pause. Take a breath. Don't let anger take control." He glances around at everyone. "Take the time to pause. Then you'll have the presence of mind to drive out of there with your BeMW."

BE A KNIGHT IN SHINING ARMOR—AND HAVE THE COURAGE TO TAKE IT OFF.

RULE NO. 3: FEEL YOUR FEELINGS AND SOFTEN THEM UP

We come to a stop outside the walls of a castle where a knight is standing guard. His armor gleams like polished silver in the afternoon sunlight. He stands taller than all of us. Looks far stronger and is formidable with his longsword and shield.

We've been here quite a while, and he hasn't moved. We ask him questions, but he gives no response.

"Is anyone really in there?" someone in the group asks.

"What if I poke him," you say.

"No." I hold up a halting hand. "Don't try and touch him. The lesson here isn't about controlling one's temper. It's about—"

A scream pierces the air, and we all turn in the direction from where it came. A horse is galloping wildly towards us, the frightened maiden riding it getting jostled in her saddle, eyes wide, hair tousled, and hanging on for dear life.

The next thing we know, the knight has dashed to the middle of the road, as if he was about to body-slam the horse to a stop. Then just as lithely and gracefully as a circus acrobat, he moves to the side, grabs hold of the horse and swings himself onto its back, landing smoothly behind the damsel in distress. Several tension-ridden seconds later, the knight is able to control the horse, slowing it down to a canter.

Behind us, the drawbridge towards the castle opens and the knight steers the horse in through the gates and they disappear inside.

As cliché, corny, and outmoded as this fairy tale character may have become, it's still a role men want to fulfill for the woman they love. Or anyone else, for that matter. Who wouldn't want to be the guy who saves the day? The one who pulls their company, a stranger, a good friend out of danger or trouble? To be a real-life knight in someone else's eyes. That's a fantasy worth fulfilling.

But here's what a lot of men may not realize. That shining armor is like a mask he puts on when he faces the world, so he never looks vulnerable and afraid. It keeps him looking unmoved by his problems while he's out fighting his daily battles. That shining armor makes him look in control. On top of his game. But that man inside? He's keeping that armor on even when he no longer needs to, so he stays protected from any attack of emotions he can't handle. Can you imagine a knight who refuses to take his armor off when he comes home to his wife at the end of the day?

That knight could be you.

A man's unconscious habit of keeping his emotional armor on may be his conscious—but ineffective—solution to keeping his partner from rocking the emotional boat. This could be a pattern those close to him would have spotted in his past relationships which started out as flings or situationships which turned into toxic, co-dependent, or emotionally unfulfilling ones in the long run. That's why it's crucial for a man to ask himself, when he's about to enter a committed relationship, if he's truly prepared to keep up the Prince Charming courtship for keeps, or is he just waiting for the time when he feels it's okay to put the armor back on?

[There are men who put their armor on again even before they "get the damsel." Meaning, he was probably unsure if she liked him, too, but didn't want to risk being vulnerable by revealing how he feels. So he pulls away and stops being "her knight" and waits to see if she'll chase him. That way, she has to put down her guard and expose her feelings first. If she doesn't go after him, he'll probably choose to let her go—without ever knowing if he broke her heart—and steel himself against the feeling of loss. I don't know how many "knights" in history gave up on finding love this way. I also don't know how many damsels' hearts were broken because a man chose to walk away rather than put away his shield.]

A man has to be honest with himself if he's really ready and willing to share more than just time, money, duties, and a bed with her if he's aiming for a happy, long-term relationship. *Do I really love her? Or do I just love having her need me—until she begins to need more than what I'm giving her now?*

This is what a man wearing an invisible armor is likely to do to keep his heart protected:

- **Stick to neutral topics:** A man ends up baffled because he engages in conversations with his partner, but she still complains about feeling a loss of connection. He doesn't realize he somehow avoids topics that involve disclosing his feelings. All the talk centers around work, household concerns, the kids, trivia, and facts about various topics of interest that only involve an exchange of opinions, not his true feelings that would matter to their relationship. She'd like to get to know the man's feelings behind the armor—if he'd let her. And she'd like him to ask about hers.

- **Not share in her emotions:** A woman shares something emotional or meaningful to her, and he gives a short reply or offers a solution to her concerns. Or he cracks a joke or teases her or offers to take her shopping to lift her spirits. Then she complains that he doesn't listen. Once again he's perplexed. "All I do is listen!" He doesn't realize that his responses instantly try to shift her away from her feelings rather than reflect how he's actively listening, absorbing her experience, and validating her feelings. What she feels is that he listens just enough so he can figure out how to "solve" her feelings like they were a problem to fix so the topic can move on. He needs to realize it's all right for her to feel sad or bad, and she'd appreciate him allowing her that space and would welcome him joining her on occasion. She has her own armor; she's not asking to borrow his.

- **Create invisible walls or -isms:** Instinctively, a man knows that being with his partner means it's going to demand that he feel his feelings. And hers. Instinctively, he'd rather not. It's possible he's avoiding negative thoughts not related to her at all. Or maybe some of them are about her too. Whether they're related to his past or the present, they're things he'd rather not deal with at the moment. So he puts up "protective measures" around him called "-isms." Workaholism, exercise-ism, alcoholism, religious-ism, gaming-ism, TV- or YouTube-ism, hobby-ism, social media-ism, so on and so forth. You get the picture. There's a whole lot of time-consuming, attention-eating, obsession-forming, and distance-setting things a man can engage in to keep himself from becoming emotionally available and vulnerable to the woman he loves. It's telling her that not only does he need his armor, but that he also needs her to keep her distance so he can just … be.

The gates to the castle courtyard open and the drawbridge lowers. Out comes the same long-haired damsel, but now on a different, much calmer horse. She's riding alone, calm and composed with a faint blush on her cheeks, her hair and gown now looking neat and pretty. If this were a fairy tale, we'd hear birds chirping and smell the essence of a flower garden in the air.

"Glad to see you're all right," you say as her horse draws near.

"Thank you, kind sir," she answers in a voice sweet as honey.

"Is the knight coming back out?" someone else asks. "We've got questions to ask. Maybe now, he'd be more open to answering."

"I'm afraid he doesn't say much. Even I can't get much out of him. He speaks more through his good deeds, you see."

"Isn't that enough?" you ask.

"I beg your pardon?" She brings the horse to a stop and looks at you.

"I mean, for you to like a man," you explain. "Isn't it enough for him to be nice and kind and good to you."

"And if he provides enough," someone else asks. "And spends time with you too."

"I suppose," she says. "That's enough for me to like him."

"*Like* him," I echo.

She looks around at all of us, calmly perched on her horse. "You're the men on a hero's quest, am I right? Aiming to fight for love so it will never die?"

The group nods in silence.

She gazes up at the castle behind the stone walls. "All the things you do to protect yourself are like bricks and mortar to a fortress that goes up around you. But you only need that while you're trying to keep the outside world from assaulting your senses. When it's time for some solitude with her, lower the drawbridge. Take off the armor. Put away the shield. True bravery for a man in love is having the courage to trust her not to hurt you."

She looks at you and says, "You're the one who asked if it's enough for a man to perform good deeds and acts of chivalry to win a woman's heart?"

You nod, and she smiles then pulls out a handkerchief from the folds of her gown. The silken cloth flies from her fingers and flutters to the ground.

You pick it up and hand it back to her. "It's yours. And you shall all receive one. Let its softness serve as a reminder that there is a price you must pay to keep a woman happy in your life."

"What's that?" you ask.

"You need to be brave enough to take off your armor and let her touch your heart. Let her feel what you feel. Otherwise, you're just another man behind a shield."

Be David against Goliath. Be bigger than your fears.

Rule No. 3: Feel Your Feelings and Soften Them Up

WE'VE COME TO THE last stop of our journey, and I've brought you to a beach covered with smooth, round pebbles. I invite you to choose one for a token to keep inside your knapsack.

I look out towards the ocean and breathe in the clean, invigorating air. Clear blue skies above. A new horizon laid out before you. It's the perfect setting for the hero you're about to meet—the mightiest one. The one I've saved till last.

"David," you say, holding up a tiny pebble between two fingers. "You consider him the mightiest?"

"After I explain why, you'll understand."

We're all afraid of getting hurt. No one ever wants to have to endure a broken heart, or to inflict pain on somebody else. So our fears, based largely on things that happened in our past or what we pessimistically predict, can lead us to do and say things or make choices we'll regret later on.

This book is dedicated to men in love. Which means, if you're reading this, quite likely, you followed your heart when you chose your partner. You chose love. You chose to fight the fear—but now you're feeling a bit of that fear again, because of the challenges your relationship is facing.

On the other hand, you might be reading this book because you suspect you're not in love but would like to be—because your partner has been good to you, and you'd like to build a happier relationship with her. Perhaps, at that time, you had begun to feel lonely being single and you rushed into a commitment. Or maybe you had to choose between the fear of being abandoned or rejected by a woman who had your heart racing versus the reassuring safety of a woman who chased you, and your brain went into fight-or-flight mode. That's when you ended up choosing not to fight for love. You gave in to your fears, went into flight mode—away from the possibility of finding the hormonal cocktail that will make your world spin. You chose the stable option. The predictable. The dependable person who won't break your heart. And now, you want to make sure that you don't break hers, because you've realized that you made the right choice.

In either scenario, there is a sincere desire in the man to make things work with his partner. And yet, why does a man in love feel the need to put his armor on? Why does he need a fortress against his emotions? Why does he turn into the Incredible Hulk in place of the mild-mannered Bruce Banner in the face of conflict? Why does he stay distant like James Bond and would rather buy her heart than bare his? He may not realize it. He may deny it. But in the depths of his soul, he's afraid of the woman he loves the most. Of losing her, disappointing her, hurting her, and being abandoned by her. It all started when he was a child, when he depended on one woman completely for sustenance, everyday care, and basic survival.

If his mother's attention was inconsistent, unreliable, or was lacking in certain ways, he would grow into an adult fearing that same sense of abandonment or neglect from his relationships.

Yet, even if in his early years, he'd received a healthy amount of caregiving, in many instances, shortly after he transitioned from being a darling baby to a little boy, his relationship with his mother changed. They had to push each other apart because he had to learn to "be a man." So he learned to bottle up his feelings, stop showing weakness, and dry his tears on his own. Then the little boy grew up to be a teenager and got his heart broken for the first time. He survived that and tried again. And again. But despite his shoulder shrugs and tipsy grins that tell the world, "I'm good," deep inside, his fears have multiplied. He now has a fear of rejection, abandonment, betrayal, failure, being shamed, becoming a burden, of losing control, or losing freedom, or not being good/rich/handsome/athletic/successful enough.

Putting them all together, that is one gigantic Goliath of fears a man needs to conquer. And yet, eventually he finds "the one" whom he chooses to marry—then maybe ends up picking up this pebble of a book because he feels lost. He believes he's doing the best he can in the relationship, but still seems to be doing nothing right.

Hopefully, now that we've gotten to this part of the book, you feel like David, coming up against the Goliath. Puny, compared to what you're up against, but armed with a little more knowledge and a better perspective so you can hit those humongous fears right between the eyes.

The hero we're talking to, the best whom I'd saved for last on this journey, is the David inside of you. A hero who stands with shoulders squared against the fears that have been manifesting in three areas: your mind, body, and heart—through your anxious thoughts, your distance-creating behavior, and your bottled-up feelings.

"Wait, what?" you ask, staggering back. "*I'm* the hero you saved for the climax?" You shake your head. "Why would you say I'm the mightiest?"

"Because you're real."

You freeze and take a gulp.

"All the heroes and icons on this journey have been symbols of ideals of men. You face real challenges. You have real fears. And you've found the courage to fight for real love." I thump the backpack hanging from your shoulders. "Now, you're equipped with what it takes to win the battle. Take a look at what you've learned along the way."

You open your Knapsack of Knowledge, and together, we go through each item and what it stands for.

- A compass to help us find our way to self-love because only then can we love another

- A detective's cap for us to keep the curiosity alive about the woman we love

- A piece of shattered rock to remind us that even the strongest among us needs a soft place to land

- A Swiss Army knife with a diamond solitaire to help us work hard at a relationship that's more than just for show

- An everlasting flower that will inspire us to keep the courtship going without end

- A BMW keychain to remind us to step on the brakes when anger strikes and steer away from negativity

- A silk handkerchief that symbolizes how soft our hearts must become for us to truly love

- A pebble that shows how any man can become a mighty warrior when he fights his fears to conquer love

Be one of the Brave Hearts. Find the courage to get close and vulnerable and allow emotional intimacy to develop; fight the fear of being abandoned, neglected, or rejected and proudly support your partner in every way. Fight the urge to keep your distance from her so you won't need to deal with whatever it is you don't want to deal with. Keeping your distance is not the way to keep the peace. Stand your ground and have those difficult conversations. Take off the armor and bare your chest to her. Show her your true feelings, instead of masking them.

You've chosen love. Now fight for it. You may feel dwarfed by these uncontrollable and gigantic feelings and fear that they will overwhelm you. Find a pebble of courage and step forward. If the fear doesn't go away, then you will have to face the moment scared.

Be like David against Goliath. Be bigger than your fears.

6

Be the Real Hero. Because Real Love is Worth Fighting For.

ONE OF SOCIETY'S MOST treasured myths is that there is only one true love for each of us to find in this lifetime. I have no data or science to prove this next theory of mine, but I believe the reason why humankind has arrived at that idealistic concept of finding "The One" is that it truly is a rarity to score a hat-trick in love. The trifecta of the mind, body, and heart—each finding a perfect match. The meeting of minds that think alike and resonate with one another. A desire to do things that demonstrate one's love that defies the passage of time. And a powerful emotional connection that fosters complete trust and openness, allowing a couple to be honest and vulnerable to one another. This "three-pronged lightning bolt" is so hard to come by, that for generations, people have come to the conclusion that true love can only strike once in a lifetime—if at all. In the modern age, it has caused great disillusionment in marriage and long-term relationships in general. One reason for this is because people keep swiping across a plethora of dating apps and fail to find even the faintest spark of something that resembles love.

That's why this myth, in some way, is the truth. When we chance upon that unique connection of mind, body, and heart—it feels like a once-in-a-lifetime thing. "The One" could really simply mean "the right one" who matches us in the most meaningful ways.

The three rules of love, in summary, are encapsulated in three simple words.

Know. Do. Feel.

Rule No. 1:   Know Who You Love—and Why

- Be Ethan Hunt. Know your mission. It's not impossible. It comes with self-acceptance and self-love.

  - Take control of your life.

  - Take stock of your core values.

  - Take charge of a change in the world.

- Be Sherlock Holmes. Ask the right questions and find the right woman.

  - Know all you can about her. Stay curious. Always.

- Be Superman to your Wonder Woman. You're both heroes with your own battles to fight.

  - Respect her. Admire her. Support her.

Rule No. 2: Do Things that Show Her You Love Her

- Be better than James Bond. Don't get a Bond Girl. Bond with your girl.

  - There are many ways a woman can feel objectified. Treat her like a lady.

- Be her Jarvis, Q, Alfred. Show her you have her back.

  - The best aphrodisiac is helping remove the brakes in her mind.

  - Find her accelerants.

- Be a Prince Charming that keeps on charming. Living happily ever after is hard work.

  - Learn to speak the language of Romance which is Thoughtfulness.

  - Be her FRIEND, by enriching your friendship through words, celebrating it with gifts, and by enjoying each other's freedom.

  - Be her LOVER, by taking care of how you present yourself, being generous with your time together, and expressing your love through eye contact and touch.

  - Be her PARTNER, by paying close attention to her needs, performing thoughtful deeds, and showing kindness.

Rule No. 3: Feel Your Feelings and Soften Them Up

- Don't be The Hulk. Don't give in to anger.

  - Drive a BeMW and steer clear of negativity.

- Be a Knight in Shining Armor—and have the courage to take it off.

  - Get rid of all your "-isms" and be emotionally naked when you're with her.

- Be David against Goliath. Be bigger than your fears.

  - Don't let her pay for fears that were put there by people in your past.

  - Fight your fears. Trust her with your heart.

I've used fictitious icons of manliness and heroism, because it's impossible to look into the private lives of real-life men and know if they truly embody what a woman wants and deserves in a relationship when nobody's looking. But I do know of one man who could rise to the challenge and become a hero for that woman in your life: You.

I'm calling on you to find the real hero inside yourself. Men and women everywhere have been victorious when it comes to love and what they and scientists have learned on how to win against the challenges, I have shared with you.

If you believe you've found "The One," go on this quest towards a deeper and greater love. Be a Brave Heart and guard what you've found—with your mind, body, and soul. Know. Do. And feel.

Love can die. Unless you fight for it.

***

Let's Build an Army of Brave Hearts

A FEW GOOD WORDS from a few good men can help spread the courage to love. If this book helped you in any way, please let others know through a review in the platform of your choice. It only takes a sentence or two to help more couples get their own chance at a happily ever after.

ACKNOWLEDGEMENTS

THIS BOOK IS AN INVITATION TO A QUEST, but it began as a personal journey of self-discovery and enlightenment. Profound gratitude and love go to my children, Alexi and Franco, who helped me navigate the tumultuous sea of emotions I was tossed into at the start of this journey. You both soothe my soul, in more ways than you can ever know, to this very day.

To Tim De Los Reyes and Vince Marquez, thank you for your priceless inputs and perspectives that added new dimensions and sparkle to my vision. What came out in the end is what I hope to be a much richer source of clarity for its readers.

To my editor, Lee McRae, thanks for your openness and valuable contributions. Beyond adding polish to the final work, your unique insights gave it more depth and breadth. A special shout-out to Katrina Yaptinchay who wrapped it all up with her cover design that captured the mission and vision perfectly.

And to my friends, clients, and relatives who've shared stories and their life's epiphanies with me through the years, my deepest thanks for giving me the honor and privilege to share your precious nuggets of wisdom with the rest of the world.

Hopefully, through this book, all your contributions combined will help make this world a happier and better place for men—and romantic couples—everywhere.

ABOUT THE AUTHOR

Cameron Draeco is a university professor, advertising executive, relationship counselor, and also the author of a series of hard science fiction books under a different pen name. In the process of writing the fourth book in the sci-fi series, which required extensive research into the dynamics of successful relationships, Draeco realized that all the information being churned up was far too valuable to be embedded in a work of fiction set in the future. Couples in romantic relationships—particularly the male half—needed all this information in the real world today.

Thus was born *Brave Hearts: 3 Rules for Men with the Courage to Love*. It's a book that finally brings into fruition a long-held dream: that a childhood passion for writing can help make this world a better place. Through this book, Draeco's hope is for romantic relationships around the world to be given a better chance at lifelong happiness.

Draeco has two "kids," who are now a medical doctor and a chef, who recently started having to deal with a constant stream of relationship advice culled from research studies—that will hopefully help them live happily ever after.

REFERENCES

1. Kardum, I., Hudek-Knezevic, J., Mehić, N., & Banov Trošelj, K. (2023). The dark triad traits and relationship satisfaction: Dyadic response surface analysis. Journal of Personality, 00, 1–17. https://doi.org/10.1111/jopy.12857

2. Eliot, L. (2021). Brain Development and Physical Aggression: How a Small Gender Difference Grows into a Violence Problem, Current Anthropology, 62 (S23), S66–78.

3. Dawson, C. (2023). Gender differences in optimism, loss aversion and attitudes towards risk, British Journal of Psychology

4. Frankenbach, J., Weber, M., Loschelder, D. D., Kilger, H., & Friese, M. (2022). Sex drive: Theoretical conceptualization and meta-analytic review of gender differences. Psychological Bulletin, 148(9-10), 621–661

5. Weinberg, M. K., Tronick, E. Z., Cohn, J. F., & Olson, K. L. (1999). Gender differences in emotional expressivity and self-regulation during early infancy. Developmental Psychology, 35(1), 175–188. https://doi.org/10.1037/0012-1649.35.1.175

6. Anderson A, Chilczuk S, Nelson K, Ruther R, Wall-Scheffler C (2023). The Myth of Man the Hunter: Women's contribution to the hunt across ethnographic contexts. PLoS ONE 18(6): e0287101. https://doi.org/10.1371/journal.pone.0287101

7. Ivan Szadvári, Daniela Ostatníková, Jaroslava Babková Durdiaková (2023). Sex differences matter: Males and females are equal but not the same, Physiology & Behavior, Volume 259, 2023, 114038, ISSN 0031-9384 https://doi.org/10.1016/j.physbeh.2022.114038.

8. Mineo, L. (2017, April 11). Good genes are nice, but joy is better. The Harvard Gazette. https://news.harvard.edu/gazette/story/2017/04/over-nearly-80-years-harvard-study-has-been-showing-how-to-live-a-healthy-and-happy-life/

9. Cox. D.A. (2021, June 29). Men's Social Circles are Shrinking, Survey Center on American Life, https://www.americansurveycenter.org/why-mens-social-circles-are-shrinking/

10. Smith, S. (2022, November 16). Why do straight men have no friends? Dazed. https://www.dazeddigital.com/life-culture/article/57460/1/straight-men-no-friends-toxic-masculinity-loneliness-u-ok

11. Kislev, E. (2019): Does Marriage Really Improve Sexual Satisfaction? Evidence From the Pairfam Data Set, The Journal of Sex Research, DOI: 10.1080/00224499.2019.1608146

12. Bombar, M. L., & Littig, L. W., Jr. (1996). Babytalk as a communication of intimate attachment: An initial study in adult romances and friendships. Personal Relationships, 3, 137–158.

13. Luterman, A. (2020, April 7). Is Baby Talk to Blame for Your (Almost) Sexless Marriage? Centre for Erotic Empathy. https://eroticempathy.ca/f/is-babytalk-to-blame-for-your-almost-sexless-marriage

14. Gladstone, J. J., Garbinsky, E. N., & Mogilner, C. (2022, March 14). Pooling Finances and Relationship Satisfaction. Journal of Personality and Social Psychology. Advance online publication. http://dx.doi.org/10.1037/pspi0000388

15. Olson, J. G., Rick, S. I, Small, D. A., Finkel, E. J. (2023). Common Cents: Bank Account Structure and Couples' Relationship Dynamics, Journal of Consumer Research, ucad020, https://doi.org/10.1093/jcr/ucad020

16. Park, L. E., Young, A. F., & Eastwick, P. W. (2015). (Psychological) Distance Makes the Heart Grow Fonder: Effects of Psychological Distance and Relative Intelligence on Men's Attraction to Women. Personality and Social Psychology Bulletin, 41(11), 1459-1473. https://doi.org/10.1177/0146167215599749

17. Xinlei (Jack) Chen, Xiaohua Zeng, Cheng Zhang (2022) Does Concealing Gender Identity Help Women Win the Competition? An Empirical Investigation into Online Video Games. Marketing Science 42(3):551-568. https://doi.org/10.1287/mksc.2022.1393

18. Miller, A. S., Byers, E. S. (2004). Actual and Desired Duration of Foreplay and Intercourse: Discordance and Misperceptions within Heterosexual Couples. The Journal of Sex Research, 41(3), 301–309. http://www.jstor.org/stable/4423787

19. Raposo, S., Rosen, N. O., & Muise, A. (2020). Self-expansion is associated with greater relationship and sexual well-being for couples coping with low sexual desire. Journal of Social and Personal Relationships, 37(2), 602-623. https://doi.org/10.1177/0265407519875217

20. Herbenick, D., Fu, T., Arter, J., Sanders, S. A., & Dodge, B. (2018). Women's Experiences with Genital Touching, Sexual Pleasure, and Orgasm: Results From a U.S. Probability Sample of Women Ages 18 to 94, Journal of Sex & Marital Therapy, 44:2, 201-212, DOI:

21. Herbenick, D., Eastman-Mueller, H., Fu, Tc. et al. Women's Sexual Satisfaction, Communication, and Reasons for (No Longer) Faking Orgasm: Findings from a U.S. Probability Sample. Arch Sex Behav 48, 2461–2472 (2019). https://doi.org/10.1007/s10508-019-01493-0

22. Constant, E., F. Vallet, J.-L. Nandrino, and V. Christophe. (2016). Personal Assessment of Intimacy in Relationships: Validity and Measurement Invariance across Gender. European Review of Applied Psychology / Revue Européenne de Psychologie Appliquée 66 (3): 109–16. doi:10.1016/j.erap.2016.04.008.

23. Hogan, J. N., Crenshaw, A. O., Baucom, K. J. W., & Baucom, B. R. W. (2021). Time Spent Together in Intimate Relationships: Implications for Relationship Functioning. Contemporary family therapy, 43(3), 226–233. https://doi.org/10.1007/s10591-020-09562-6

24. Selcuk, E., Karagobek, A.B., Gunaydin, G. (2018). Responsiveness as a Key Predictor of Happiness: Mechanisms and Unanswered Questions. In: Demir, M., Sümer, N. (eds) Close Relationships and Happiness across Cultures. Cross-Cultural Advancements in Positive Psychology, vol 13. Springer, Cham. https://doi.org/10.1007/978-3-319-89663-2_1

25. Williams, B. Scientific Impact of Kindness Pt. 1. Think Kindness. https://thinkkindness.org/all-things-kindness/scientific-impact-of-kindness-pt-1/

26. Azil, A., Bennett, B., Nadeau, M., and Zucker, J. (2019). Making it Work: How Dual-career Couples find Career Fulfillment. McKinsey & Company Report.

27. Petriglieri, J. (2019, September-October). How Dual-Career Couples Make It Work. Harvard Business Review.

28. O'Leary, K. D., Acevedo, B. P., Aron, A., Huddy, L, and Mashek, D. (2012). Is Long-Term Love More than a Rare Phenomenon? If So, What are Its Correlates. Social Psychological and Personality Science DOI: 10.1177/1948550611417015 2012 3: 241

29. Acevedo, B. P., Aron, A., Fisher, H.E., Brown, L. L.. (2012) Neural correlates of long-term intense romantic love, Social Cognitive and Affective Neuroscience, Volume 7, Issue 2, February 2012, Pages 145–159, https://doi.org/10.1093/scan/nsq092

30. The Mind of a Man. WebMD. https://www.webmd.com/women/features/mind-of-man

31. Holmen, J., Langballe, E., Midthjell, K., Holmen, T., Fikseaunet, A., Saltvedt, I., Tambs, K. (2013) Gender differences in subjective memory impairment in a general population: the HUNT study, Norway. BMC Psychology; 1 (1): 19 DOI: 10.1186/2050-7283-1-19

32. Baumeister, R. & Catanese, K., & Vohs, K. (2001). Is There a Gender Difference in Strength of Sex Drive? Theoretical Views, Conceptual Distinctions, and a Review of Relevant Evidence. Personality and Social Psychology Review - PERS SOC PSYCHOL REV. 5. 242-273. 10.1207/S15327957PSPR0503_5.

33. Rauer, A., Sabey, A. K., Proulx, C. M., Volling, B. L. (2019). What are the Marital Problems of Happy Couples? A Multimethod, Two-Sample Investigation. Family Process, 2019; DOI: 10.1111/famp.12483

34. Seager, C. (2016, October 6) My career discovering the secret to everlasting love: "I just fell into it." The Guardian. https://www.theguardian.com/careers/2016/oct/06/my-career-discovering-the-secret-to-everlasting-love-i-just-fell-into-it

Made in the USA
Columbia, SC
11 April 2024

b54142db-d833-4f4a-9192-5c73dabbfec6R01